MW00738136

THE JEWELRY DESIGN SOURCE BOOK

THE JEWELRY DESIGN SOURCE BOOK

PATRICIA BAYER · VIVIENNE BECKER · HELEN CRAVEN · PETER HINKS · RONALD LIGHTBOWN ·

JACK OGDEN · DIANA SCARISBRICK

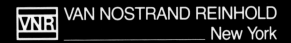
VAN NOSTRAND REINHOLD
New York

Published in the U.S.A. by
Van Nostrand Reinhold
115 Fifth Avenue
New York, New York 10003

This book was designed and produced by
Quarto Publishing plc
The Old Brewery
6 Blundell Street
London N7 9BH

Consultant editor Diana Scarisbrick

Project editor Henrietta Wilkinson
Editor Mary Chesshyre
Designer Hazel Edington
Picture researcher Deirdre O'Day

Editorial director Carolyn King
Art director Moira Clinch

Typeset in Great Britain by Pearl Graphics, London
Ampersand, Bournemouth and QV Typesetting

Manufactured in Hong Kong by Regent Publishing Services Ltd
Printed by Leefung-Asco Printers Ltd, Hong Kong

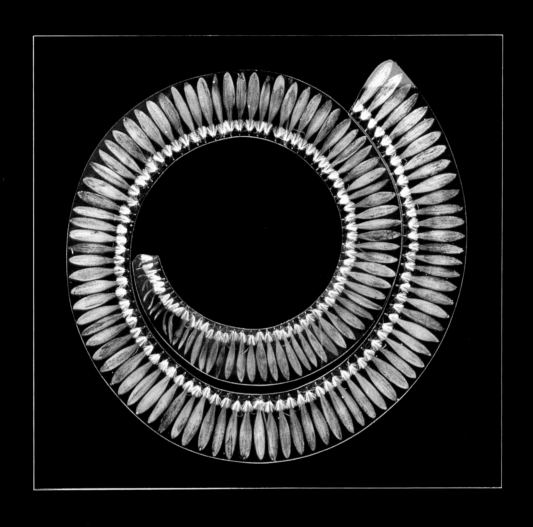

CONTENTS

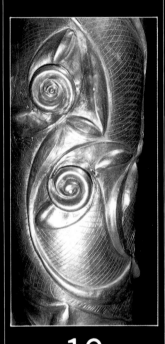
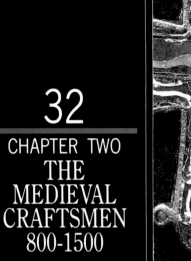
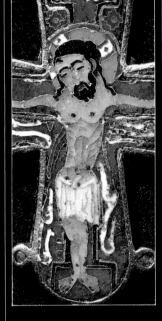
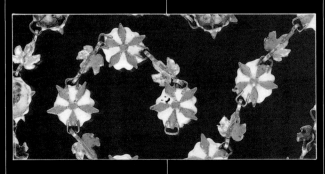
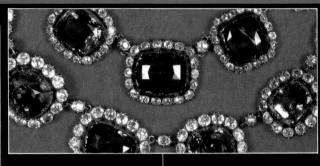
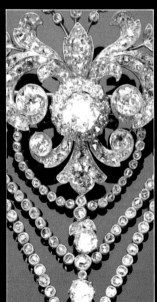

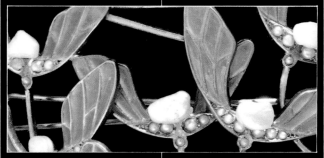
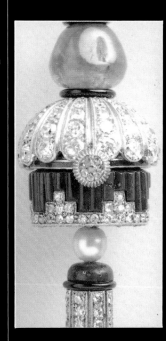
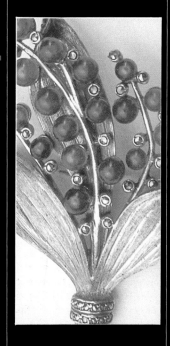
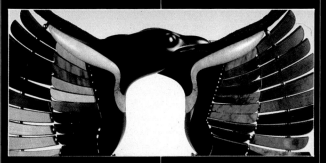

INTRODUCTION

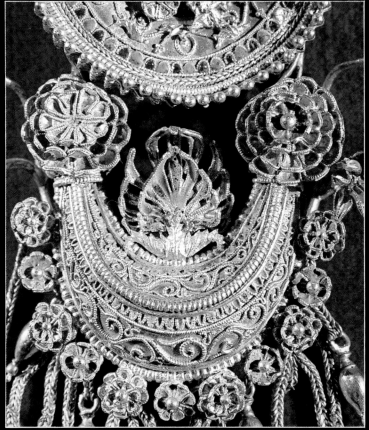

The ancient goldsmith's mastery of the techniques of enameling and filigree is demonstrated in this detail from a gold jewel for the forehead. The crescent, which hangs from a round disk, terminates in rosettes at each end, and from it hang smaller rosettes and plaited gold chains. The enameled gold honeysuckle in the center is a classical motif often executed in diamonds by jewelers of the late 19th and early 20th centuries.

The story of jewelry over seven thousand years of civilization covers the response of successive generations of craftsmen and women to the challenge of fashioning rare and precious materials into personal ornaments which express the prevailing artistic style.

This rich and diverse panorama begins in the ancient world, when the basic techniques of the goldsmith were mastered at an astonishingly early date. Outstanding achievements came from the Etruscans, who brought filigree and granulation techniques to a peak of perfection never since equaled, and from the Hellenistic court jewelers who mastered the art of modeling human figures for earrings, necklaces, and bracelets bright with red garnets and enamel. Sometimes there were marked changes of style: the luxurious Roman gold ornaments laden with green emeralds and shining white pearls contrast sharply with the barbaric, powerful polychrome jewels of the Dark Ages, which followed the end of the Empire.

An entirely new note was struck in the Middle Ages, when jewels expressed the ideals of Christianity and chivalry in the language of the cathedral builders with crockets and canopied niches. Another high point was attained in the classical climate of the Renaissance, when goldsmiths created elaborate compositions highlighted with enamels and gemstones. This figurative style vanished in the next phase, when the reign of the gem-setter began and the contribution of the goldsmith declined progressively, as jewels became no more than a vehicle for the display of gemstones and artistry was subordinated to a concern with intrinsic value. In the rococo period the trend toward lightness and asymmetry resulted in less dense and more open designs which adapted elegantly to the severe outlines of the Neo-classical style current from the 1770s.

A Taste for Opulence

The complex course of 19th-century developments begins with the grandiose jewels that were created for the court of the Emperor Napoleon and which set the standard for the rest of Europe long after the defeat at Waterloo in 1815. At the same time emerged Romanticism, a movement inspired by nostalgia for the picturesque world of the Middle Ages and Renaissance. Around

1850, Romanticism merged with a strong current of Revivalism embracing the whole of history and leading to the recreation of the gold ornaments of antiquity and the Dark Ages for daytime wear. The growing taste for luxury, encouraged by prosperity, low taxation, and a hierarchical social system, was expressed by increasingly opulent displays of diamonds after the discovery of mines in South Africa in the 1860s. This event transformed the character of jewelry which for several decades concentrated on glitter and sparkle rather than on color, design, and the expression of ideas. At the turn of the century, however, there was a two-fold reaction against the banality of so much diamond jewelry. First, Cartier and Boucheron adopted a new style, of 18th-century inspiration, comprising trelliswork and garlands of stylized flowers, using platinum for settings. This diamond jewelry epitomizes the gracious elegance of the Belle Epoque.

At around the same time, the Art Nouveau jewelers, led by René Lalique, created a great stir at the Paris Exhibition of 1900 with designs taken directly from nature and executed in materials such as horn and ivory, chosen for their aesthetic quality rather than intrinsic value. Although beautiful as works of art, they were not suited for practical purposes, and the style disappeared – as did the garland style – with the outbreak of the First World War. Soon after the peace of 1918 came jewels in the Art Deco style, which owed nothing to tradition and little to nature, but instead was closely associated with contemporary art – Cubism and Abstractionism – and the streamlined architecture of the Bauhaus, softening only in the mid-1930s when figurative and floral motifs were re-introduced by Cartier.

Fine jewelry after the Second World War was adapted to the taste of a clientele buying for investment as well as for show. The emphasis was on the quality of the stones, perfectly faceted, and mounted in streamlined flexible settings in tune with current couture fashion. Simultaneously, all over the world, artist jewelers were emerging both for the design and execution of jewels, often selling direct to clients. This movement, which stems from the 19th-century Arts and Crafts tradition, has recently been affected by the high cost of precious stones and metal, leading to experiments with cheap materials such as plastic.

The Virgin and Child, favorite theme of medieval sculpture was also interpreted by jewelers in gold, enameled in the round. This group probably came from a morse, or large brooch designed to fasten a priest was chasuble when officiating at the altar.

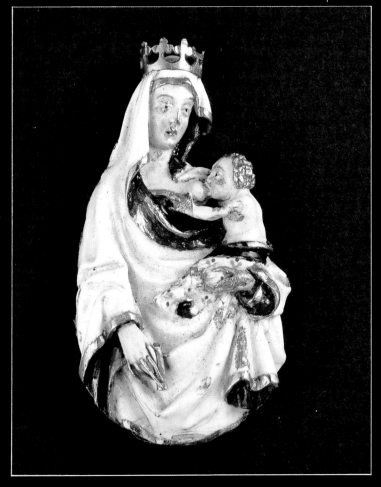

INTRODUCTION

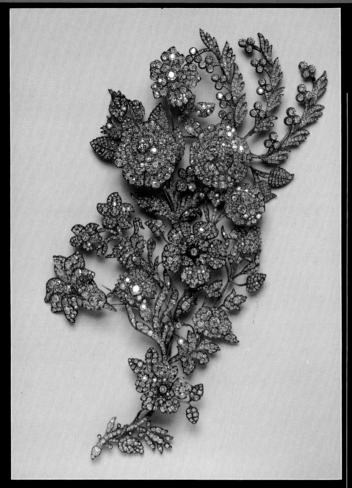

A love of flowers and leaves has inspired jewelers throughout history. Mid-19th-century taste demanded botanical jewels glittering with diamonds and large in scale, like this bouquet of carnations and roses. Some of the flowers are mounted on trembler springs for additional glitter.

The Supremacy of the Parisian Jewelers

Amid so much diversity some factors have remained constant for long periods, notably the supremacy of Paris. Since 1200–1400, when the Parisian jewelers were regarded as pre-eminent in design and craftsmanship, this lead has, for the most part, been maintained. French designs were diffused abroad in engraved editions of pattern books published from the 16th to the 19th centuries, while practical expertise emigrated with Huguenot craftsmen after the Revocation of the Edict of Nantes in 1685. Other jewelers were invited to work at the courts of foreign rulers, and visiting ladies took advantage of their time in Paris to have their jewels reset. Although the French Revolution of 1789 brought this luxury trade to a standstill, it was triumphantly revived under Napoleon. Even the collapse of the Second Empire in 1870 could not shake it. The great dynasties of Cartier, Boucheron, and Chaumet survived the disaster unscathed and expanded their empires into the 20th century, setting up branches in London, New York, Switzerland, and Japan. It was from Paris, too, that the pioneers of Art Nouveau and Art Deco emerged to generate the ideas which the great jewelers then transformed into fashionable jewels. As a result of the close connection between the leading jewelers and couture houses, designs have been conceived in harmony with the latest fashions in dress; this has contributed to the continuing success of the French firms in the post-Second World War period.

Whereas some motifs, such as snakes, appear only intermittently in the long history of jewelry, others have been continually reinterpreted. The flowers and leaves ornamenting Hellenistic diadems also decorate the shoulders of medieval rings, are enameled on the covers of 17th-century lockets and watch-cases, and, studded with diamonds and colored stones, appear as asymmetrical bouquets for the 18th-century lady to pin in her hair or on her bodice. At the 1878 International Exhibition, the stand of the Parisian jeweler O. Massin attracted great crowds who came to stare at his diamond botanical jewelry, which, mounted on trembler springs, captured the grace and lightness of the living flower. One of the great achievements of 20th-century jewelry has been the interpretation of floral designs in the exacting "invisible setting" technique introduced by Van Cleef & Arpels in 1936.

Jewels as Love Tokens

Jewels are the most prized of all love tokens, and motifs expressing sentiment have a long history: hands clasped in trust, Cupid's arrows, gimmel rings with twin hoops and bezels symbolic of the married state, lockets containing the hair and miniatures of loved ones. Whereas these are not acceptable to 20th-century taste, the heart, which first appears in medieval jewelry, and then – jeweled or enameled, single, twinned, wounded, flying or crowned– in all successive periods, maintains its appeal today.

Cameos and intaglios have also seen successive revivals. In antiquity they were valued above all other precious objects, and those that descended to medieval princes were likewise mounted in richly jeweled settings of which the Schaffhausen Onyx is the most celebrated. The difficult art of gem engraving was practiced again in the Renaissance, when hat badges, pendants, necklaces, rings, and bracelets were set with cameos and intaglios representing mythological divinities, the heroes of classical history, and ancient and modern illustrious men and women. In the 18th century Madame de Pompadour– herself a gifted engraver - brought engraved hardstones back into fashion for jewelry, and demand in the Neoclassical period was so great that it could be met only by Josiah Wedgwood's ceramic reproductions. Throughout the 19th century, cameos were favorite form of daytime jewel, signifying both high culture and the experience of travel, for the best source was the workshops of Rome, heirs to a tradition going to the Roman Empire.

Unlike their settings, engraved hardstones have escaped the fate of recycling, and so it is possible to follow the development of this art throughout its history. This is not the case with jewelry, which is almost always doomed as it passes from one generation to the next for resetting according to the latest fashion. Thus, what has come down to us only represents a small part of a much wider picture, and the objects illustrated in this book provide only a hint of the glorious creations of the jewelers of past times.

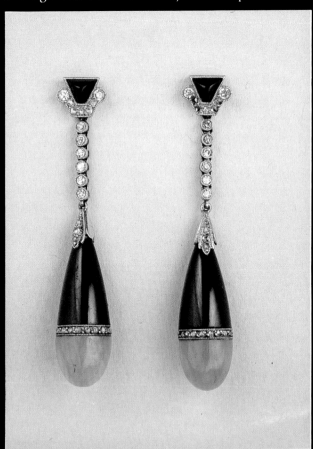

The supremacy of the French jeweler, which began in the early 13th century, has been maintained ever since, with the exception of a few brief periods. Talent may pass down through several generations, as in the firm of Boucheron, which made these striking jade, onyx, and diamond earrings, c. 1924. Founded in 1858 it is at the center of an empire which now extends to Japan.

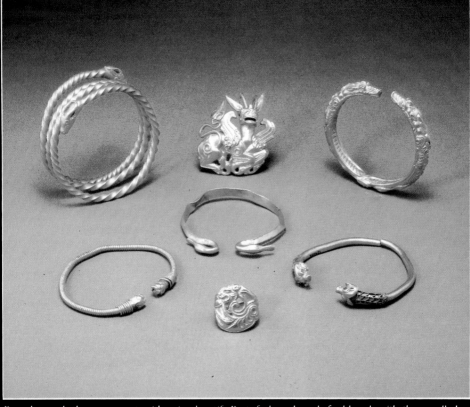

Bracelets and other ornaments with animal motifs. Part of a large hoard of goldwork with the so-called Oxus treasure, from the 5th-3rd centuries BC, found over one hundred years ago in Afghanistan.

CHAPTER · ONE

THE ANCIENT WORLD

Cast and hammered gold

·

Egypt and Mesopotamia

·

Greeks and Romans

·

The influence of Christendom

·

The Dark Ages

JACK OGDEN

INTRODUCTION

The Age of Gold was a legendary, Utopian period early in man's history. It is aptly described. Gold occurs naturally in the earth in an attractive ready-to-use state, and so was one of the first metals ever used. The softness of gold meant that it had a greater ornamental than functional value; it was the color of the sun; and it was not affected by corrosion and decay. The beauty of gold, in the eyes of early man, meant that it was frequently singled out as a fitting gift for the gods or a suitable accompaniment for the dead. Its unalterability, in chemical terms, supported such human desires and ensured that gold artefacts from the earliest periods could survive in near pristine condition.

The concept of jewelry is timeless. People have always had an instinctive desire to adorn themselves. Simple ornaments of berries, soft stones, animal teeth, and the like date back to the Stone Age, as do some simple gold objects. However, the construction of jewelry from gold or silver, and the combination of these with colored stones, really began in earnest around the beginning of the Bronze Age. So, in the ancient Near East, gold and colored-stone jewelry is rare in burials much before about 3000 BC; In Western Europe, a gold jewelry industry was flourishing soon after 2500 BC.

The Old World has thus seen a production of gold jewelry for some 5,000 years with a continuous development in designs and techniques. Designs reflect all aspects of the societies in which they blossomed. Religion, superstition, social organization, economics, trade, and warfare all played a part. As new techniques were introduced, new decorative ideas were possible and new materials, such as harder stones or colored glasses and enamel, could be incorporated.

Gold and can easily be hammered out into thin sheets, so ancient gold jewelry was usually made from thin sheet gold. Cast gold ornaments were unusual except in certain regions, such as Western Europe. Ancient gold was made with a minimum assortment of tools, and these were simply made from metal, wood, or bone.

By about 2000 BC, the goldsmiths in the Near East had developed the skills necessary to form, manipulate, and join very small components. The ultimate expression of this skill was the technique of granulation, which spread rapidly through the Eastern Mediterranean and the Near East. Granulation work consists of designs of minute gold spheres each of which can be well under .02 in (.5mm) in diameter. Much of the earliest wire filigree and granulation work is, however, not particularly fine, which can give a somewhat barbaric appearance to the jewelry.

The combination of colored stones with gold was popular in Egypt and Mesopotamia from an early period. Carnelian and lapis lazuli were the favorites, but green feldspar and other stones were also employed. In Europe the fashion seems to have been for gold alone, and here colored stones were seldom set in gold much before the Roman period.

Extensive trade contacts meant that there was a general constancy in the techniques and materials used in jewelry making throughout the Near East. With jewelry designs, however, more localized characteristics are identifiable. In most parts of the Old World, the designs are essentially abstract, geometric, or organic in form. We find spirals, circles, rosettes, and fruit-like fluted beads, timeless forms that can be paralleled in most parts of the world and in all

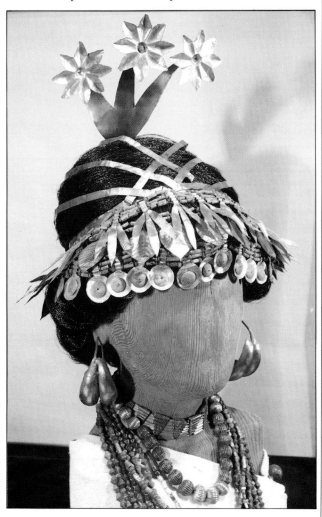

periods. The only civilization that stands out in contrast is Egypt: strongly representational forms were very much a characteristic of Egyptian, jewelry, which could quite literally spell out meanings in its designs. In most other parts of the Old World, from Ireland to Persia, such obviously representational designs were for long the exception rather than the rule. We can think of much Egyptian jewelry as icons in which colored stones take the place

Lapis lazuli and carnelian are combined with gold (and a little silver) in these Sumerian ornaments from Ur, which date from around 2500 BC. These were the favorite stones in early Near Eastern jewelry. The simple but strong shapes of the beads and earrings alongside the stylized gold flower-heads and leaves, accent the timeless majesty of these early court jewels.

of pigment and such frippery as granulation work is rarely found. This representational approach has its parallel in the strictly defined pictorial hieroglyphics of written Egyptian, which contrasts with, say, the abstract, wedge-like cuneiform writing of Mesopotamia.

In the gold jewelry produced by the Minoan and Mycenaean civilizations in Greece, Crete, and Cyprus the emphasis is again on goldwork rather than stones, though rudimentary enamelwork is found – perhaps its earliest occurrence in the world. Egyptian influence in some Mycenaean jewelry is obvious, but there are also links with Western Asia and Northern Europe. The Mycenaeans wore gold seal rings and earrings. Signet rings had been known in Egypt since around 2000 BC, but were never a characteristic of Western Asia, whereas the Egyptians, for some unfathomable reason, did not wear earrings prior to about 1500 BC., one thousand years after their Mesopotamian counterparts had first worn them. Egyptian rings were initially seals – usually the seal took the form of an oval representation of the scarab beetle, the flat base of which was engraved with a design that could be used to make seal impressions. In Western Asia the traditional seal type was an engraved cylinder that could be rolled over clay to leave an impression. Such seals were not well suited to setting in rings but were better worn as pendants.

The Iron Age

Soon after 1000 BC we see a wind of change in jewelry designs, except in Egypt with its all-pervading conservatism. The new styles came from and were spread by the Phoenicians, while the increase in the degree of precision and repetition of techniques might well reflect the new availability of iron tools. It is somewhat ironic that the Phoenician style was, ultimately, Egyptian in origin, but, newly interpreted and with an accent on granulation and other fine decorative techniques, it spread around the Mediterranean from Syria to Spain. The superb, delicate jewelry of the Etruscans, for example, best known for its minuscule and perfect granulation work, owes much of its inspiration to the Phoenicians and is very closely related in technical terms.

As the Phoenicians traveled the Mediterranean world, other influences were having an effect to the east and north. Animal motifs, perhaps originating in the southern steppes of Russia, spread down into Turkey and Persia and emerged in ornaments such as bracelets and torques with animal-head terminals. As the Persian Empire grew, a variety of motifs, styles, techniques, and even craftsmen intermixed over a vast region. Farther west the Celtic floral and animal styles appeared, perhaps filtering across from the same Russian steppes. The Celtic forms, to which Art Nouveau would look more than 2000 years later, give a contradictory feeling of freedom combined with a sense of mysterious secrecy. This European Celtic style passed into

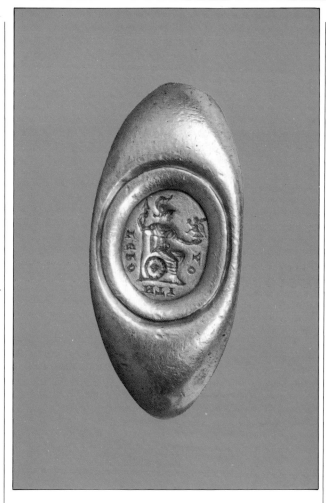

As the Roman period progressed, men often aspired to wear as many gold rings as their fingers and purses could bear. The rise of a large middle class, with access to gold (in the form of coins), greatly widened the market for jewelry. The ring shown here has a gold bezel delicately chiseled with a figure of the goddess Roma being offered a victor's wreath by a small winged Victory. The inscription tells us that the original owner was named Gerontius. This ring was found with other jewelry at Tarsus, in Syria, and dates to around AD 300.

Anglo-Saxon, Viking, and other Dark Age jewelry.

As the Persian Empire gradually fell to Alexander the Great from 334 BC, the homogenization of Near Eastern jewelry became almost complete. Even in conservative Egypt, Hellenism prevailed: initially the Egyptian and Greek traditions in jewelry co-existed, but then the age-old Egyptian forms were superseded almost entirely by cosmopolitan Hellenistic styles.

Greek jewelry of this period is characterized by its abundant applied decoration, most typically fine filigree arranged in the form of spirals, waves, and floral sprays. It is less self-absorbed in intricacy than Etruscan work, and granulation was employed mainly to highlight or punctuate the filigree work. The filigree itself was very frequently embellished with enamel, but unfortunately the ravages of time have meant that Hellenistic jewelry is seldom seen today in its full polychrome splendor. Blood-red garnets were the most popular stones in Hellenistic jewelry, though by the 2nd century BC emeralds, pearls and sometimes onyxes were also popular.

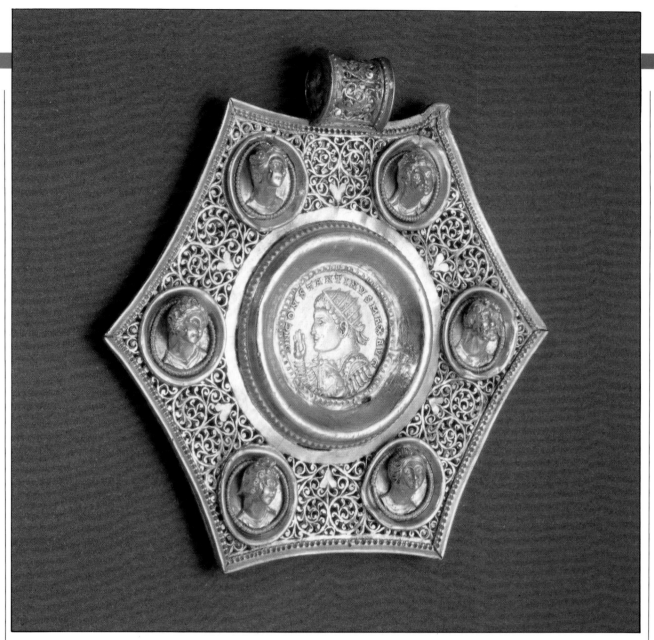

Gold jewelry set with coins became popular toward the end of the 3rd century AD. In many cases it could have been a gift – perhaps a betrothal exchange or a presentation from the Emperor to a favored subject. This magnificent pendant of delicate chisel-pierced openwork is embellished with high busts of mythological figures and is set with a double solidus minted in AD 321.

Rome, Byzantium, and the West

In the Near East, particularly in Syria, the Hellenistic taste for lavish decoration continued into the early centuries of the Christian Era, but in Italy a more severe, Roman style of jewelry came into existence. Gone is the fiddly precision and fear of open spaces of Etruscan goldwork. In its place we have a love of stronger and starker forms such as the bracelets and earrings composed of simple burnished gold hemispheres. Where colored stones are used pearls and emeralds reign supreme, not the bright red garnets and polychrome enamels of the Hellenistic world.

Paradoxical as it might seem, we have very little Roman jewelry from Italy, apart from the large quantity of ornaments from Pompeii and the neighboring towns devastated by the eruption of Vesuvius in AD 79. Most surviving Roman–period jewelry appears elsewhere in the Roman Empire. Much is from Asia Minor, Syria, and the Levant. This jewelry is supplemented by finds from Europe, which establish the overall unity of Roman jewelry. As the Roman period progressed the trend was away from the starker Italian Roman forms and back toward the Hellenistic tradition with its love of ornamentation and colored stones.

With the spread of Christianity through the Roman Empire in the early 4th century AD, Christian iconography superseded, or, in many cases, adapted, pagan Roman and Hellenistic designs. Colored stones were popular, particularly emeralds, pearls, and sapphires. When the real stones were not available glass substitutes were used –with or without the knowledge of the buyer. There was a love of intricate goldwork, particularly the pierced openwork which gives lace-like lattices of gold. Gold coins began to be worn set in rings and hanging from pendants. All this early Byzantine jewelry provided outward signs of wealth and affluence which appalled the early Christian Fathers.

Christianity itself added a new repertoire of motifs, but that did not mean the loss of earlier traditions. For example, when we see Byzantine rings with bezels in the form of lotus flowers – which had become a symbol of the Virgin Mary and Christ's birth – we are also looking at the age-old Egyptian symbol of the lotus as the birthplace of the young sun god.

History books usually tell us that with the demise of the Roman Empire Europe was plunged into the Dark Ages for half a millennium before re-emerging in the dawn of the Medieval period. The jewelry historian knows how untrue this is. Jewelry produced by the Saxons, Merovingians, Franks, Ostrogoths, Vikings, and others compares favorably with anything produced before or since, in terms of both design and technical ability. The goldsmith's craft continued, without a harsh break, from the Ancient to the Medieval world, forever building on, and adapting, the designs and concepts of earlier jewelers.

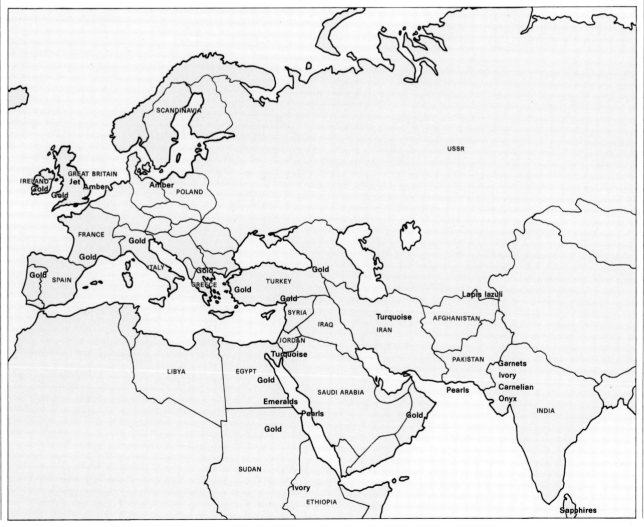

A modern map indicating some of the major gold and gem sources of the ancient world. Different gemstones were favored at different periods; for example, emeralds and pearls were widely used only from the Hellenistic period onward, and sapphires were seldom worn before Roman times.

INFLUENCES

Following the adoption of the Christian faith by the Eastern Roman Empire in the early 4th-century AD, jewelers and other artists adapted and combined both Christian and pre-Christian iconography. In many cases, iconographic continuation was possible by reinterpreting earlier concepts in Christian terms.

In Christian art the lily or lotus flower was a symbol of the Virgin Mary. This 7th-century ring (**1**), has a bezel in the form of a lotus flower, and its allusion to the Virgin Mary is strengthened by the pierced inscription on the shank, by which the wearer appeals to the protection of the Theotokos (the Mother Of God).

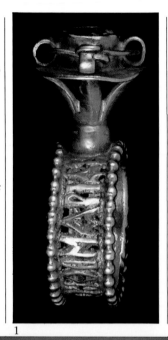

1

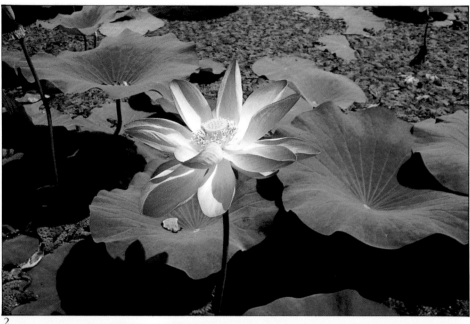

2

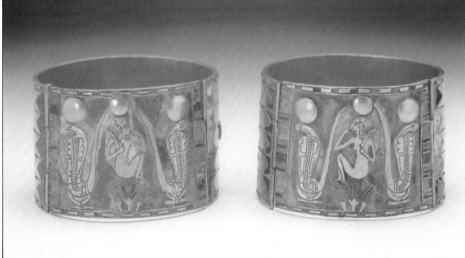

3

In ancient Egyptian mythology the young young sun god, Horus, came forth from the lotus flower. Looking at a lotus (**2**), which opens to the sun each morning, we can understand how such a legend began. In Egyptian art we see representations of the young sun god appearing from a lotus. The pair of gold bracelets (**3**), dating from about 940 BC, show the birth of the sun god with flanking uraeus serpents – the protectors of royalty – a highly suitable design for the original wearer who was a son of a Pharaoh. The bracelets were inlaid with lapis lazuli and blue glass, although much of the inlay is now missing.

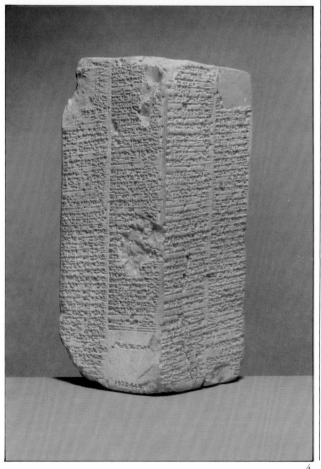

4

The Egyptian hieroglyphic script shown (**5**) is from the temple of Kom Ombo. The necklet from the tomb of Tutankhamun (**6**) combines a variety of symbols. The main pendant shows the eye of Horus flanked by the Royal Protectors. The counter-balance is composed of two symbols, helping the general welfare of the wearer. Art was representational and thus could be "read."

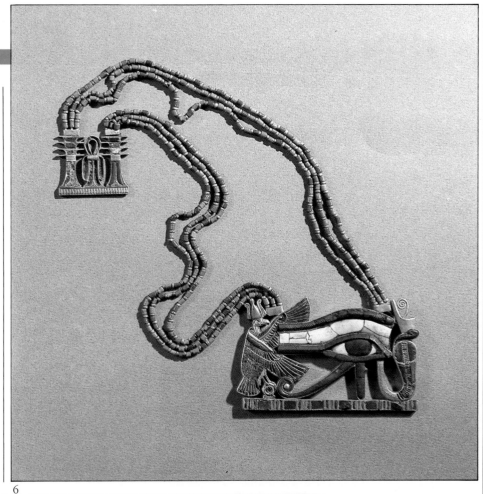

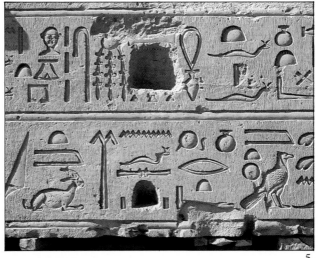

5 6

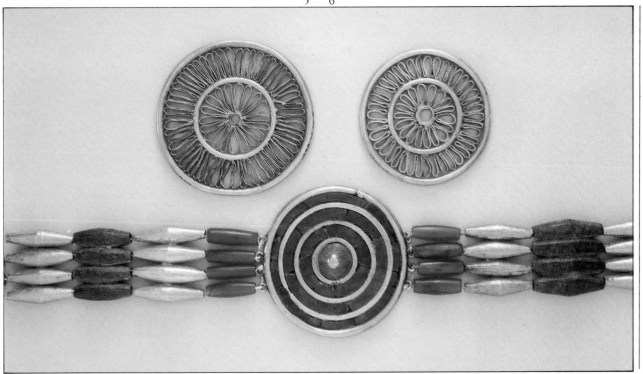

7

In Egyptian art there was an overall unity of proportions and motifs, whereas in Western Asia there was a less formal canon, and art was thus not so obviously readable. The Sumerian necklet and ornamental disks from Ur (**7**) (c.2500 BC) cannot be compared with, or interpreted in comparison with, the wedge-like cuneiform writing seen here impressed into a Sumerian clay tablet (**4**). What we see as abstraction in both writing and jewelry designs must reflect something of the underlying society. This is also true of the formal pictorial nature of Egyptian writing and has a close connection to the set repertoire of Egyptian jewelry motifs.

GOLD IN THE BRONZE AGE

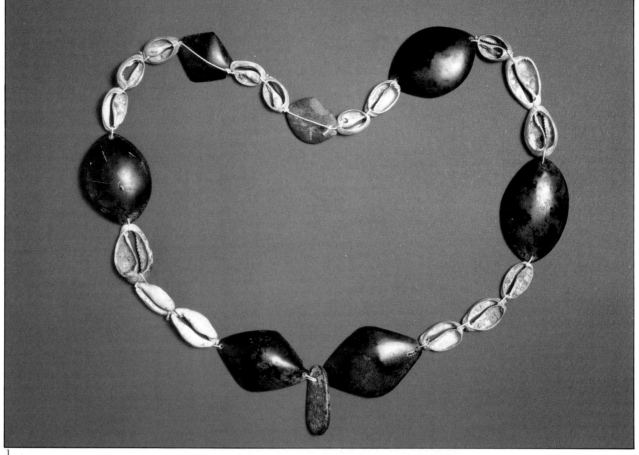

The use of shells, as in this 7,000-year-old necklace from Arpachiya, in what is now Iraq (**1**), dates back to time immemorial. The sliced cowrie shells were originally filled with a red substance which would have contrasted with the shiny black obsidian beads. Obsidian beads are hard to cut and polish, and their maker saved time and effort by leaving the backs unpolished. The black bead, top center, is of mud, not obsidian. The original thread, which has since disappeared, would have been of organic fiber or, perhaps, animal hair.

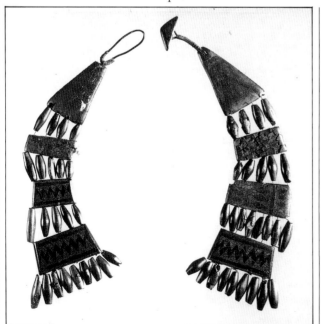

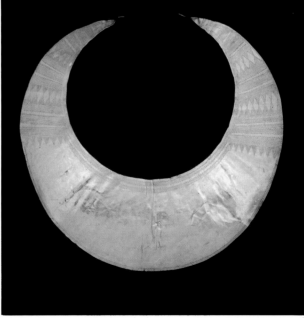

Designs and concepts can often transcend the nature of the materials used. We can see this in the similar overall forms of the jet necklace from Scotland (**2**) and the gold collar from Ireland (**3**). Both date from around 1800–1500 BC and have strictly geometric ornamentation.

In keeping with its age and Western European origin, the gold collar is formed from a single piece of hammered gold sheet. The decoration is incised or scored, a process rarely seen in Eastern Mediterranean goldwork of the Bronze Age.

THE EARLY JEWELERS

Our knowledge of the earliest jewelers is gleaned from pictorial and literary evidence. Reliefs in Egyptian tombs show all aspects of the craft from the basic recovery of the raw materials, through the working methods, to the finished articles being displayed, recorded, and weighed. Texts refer to important men bearing a variety of titles connected with the supervision of the goldsmith's craft. The craftsmen under their control, depicted bent over their anvils or drilling stone beads, are anonymous.

A glimpse of the lives of the individual craftsmen is better obtained from the less formal texts of Western Asia. These include inventories listing all types of jewelry. We also learn about the administration of the workshops, the types of precious stones and their origins, and the numbers of craftsmen; and,

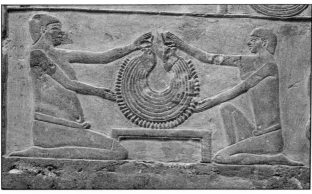

A detail from a relief in the tomb of Mereruka at Saqqara, Egypt, showing two craftsmen with a newly made necklet, c. 2300 BC.

possibly we hear of itinerant craftsmen.

A recent, remarkable discovery at Larsa, in Iraq, was a sealed jar dating from 1738 BC, which contained jewelers' tools, weights, gold jewelry, lapis lazuli and other stones, scrap silver, and, most interestingly, a seal bearing the name of the original owner. The jar was found in what

had been his workshop. This is so far the only occurrence from the ancient world of evidence of a named jeweler, the site of his workshop, his tools, and specimens of his handiwork.

The workshop of this named jeweler was situated in a temple; and, indeed, most of the jewelers of which we have a record were connected with a temple or a

court. The circulation of gold, silver, and valuable gemstones was for long controlled by temple or state.

Whether working for temple or for court, or plying his trade among the richer members of society, the ancient goldsmith used remarkably few and unsophisticated tools. Nevertheless, with skill and time at his disposal he was able to produce exquisite jewelry which has not only withstood the test of time but also acted as an inspiration to jewelers in recent centuries.

The fine necklace (4) with its elaborate and precise granulation work was supposedly found at Dilbat in Iraq. On the basis of the technique used and the style of some of the elements, the necklet can be dated to c. 1700 BC. The pair of figures on the sides probably represent the goddess Lama.

The granulation work and the fluted sheet-gold beads have parallels in other gold jewelry from Iraq and Syria and show the high levels of workmanship, and basic homogeneity, of the jewelry of the period.

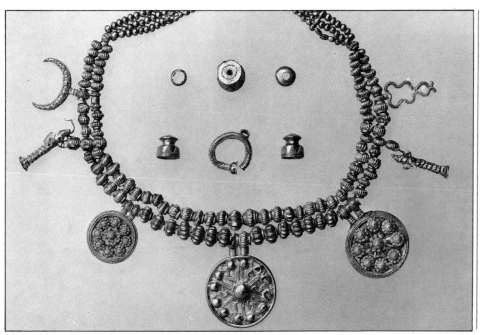

4

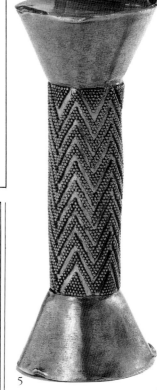

5

The geometric form of the gold pendant (5) contrasts with the representational nature of most jewelry from ancient Egypt. The pendant would have originally contained a charm of some sort. A date of c. 1900–1800 BC puts the fine granulation work among the earliest known from Egypt.

GOLD IN THE BRONZE AGE

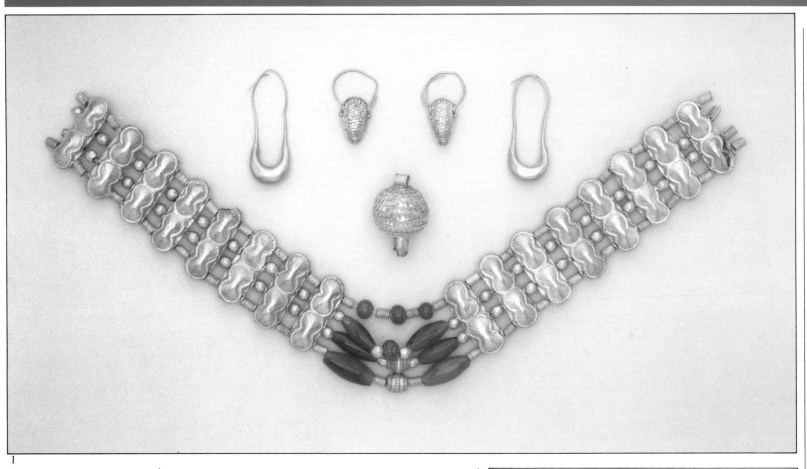

1

The two pairs of earrings, pendant and necklace (**1**) were all excavated in 1896 at the site of Enkomi, in Cyprus. They date from the Mycenaean period, around 1400–1300 BC.

The geographical position of the island of Cyprus laid it open to influences from Egypt, Western Asia, and the Aegean. The goldwork shown here, however, is entirely Cypriot. The long drop-hoop earrings of hollow sheet gold and the ear hoops with embossed, highly stylized bull-head pendants, are most typically Cypro-Mycenaean. The necklet, composed of gold shield-like motifs, spherical and spiral gold beads and carnelian beads, might harken back to foreign concepts, but it is a fine version of another favored Cypriot ornament.

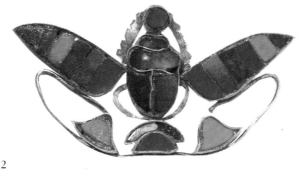

2

The little gold sphere pendant represents a pomegranate and has a minute, repetitive triangle design in granulation.

The Egyptian scarab beetle, symbol of the sun and creation, was a popular motif. This winged scarab, inlaid with colored stones and faience (**2**), dates from c. 1885 BC. The scarab clasps the sun, and as in so much Egyptian

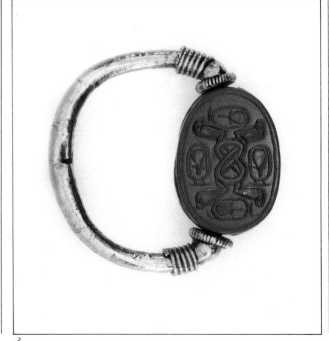

3

jewelry, the motifs shown spell out a name in hieroglyphs – in this case one name of King Sesostris II. The wing span is only 1½ in (3.5 cm).

Scarabs were also mounted in rings, their bases engraved to be used as seals. The gold and green jasper example (**3**) dates from around 1500 BC.

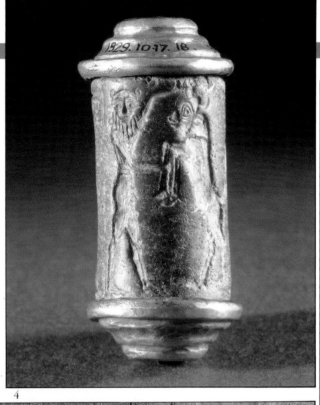

Unlike the Egyptian scarab seal, the traditional cylinder-shaped seal from Western Asia was usually too large to be worn set in a ring. The usual way of carrying a cylinder seal was as a pendant. The very fine lapis lazuli mounted in gold was excavated at Ur, in modern Iraq, on the skeleton of an obviously important man (**4**). He also had gold bracelets, a necklet and other jewelry, all dating from c. 2100 BC.

4

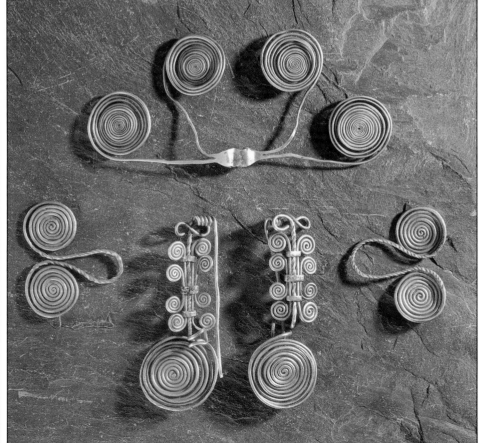

5

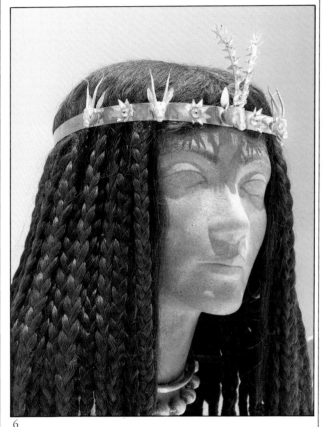

6

The earliest European jewelry was usually made from one piece of gold. For separate components, rivets or folds were used, not soldering. This was also almost universally true of bronze jewelry. The gold spiral jewelry from Hungary (**5**), of about 1000 BC, illustrates this simple construction. The jewelry consists of gold sheet hammered into wires and coiled to form brooches, pendants, and a pectoral or diadem.

Jewelry from Egypt and Western Asia stands out in contrast to this with its expert use of soldering to join separate and often miniscule components. The diadem with star and gazelle motifs (**6**), found in the Egyptian Delta, combines a simple design with delicate workmanship. The form is more Western Asiatic than Egyptian in style and might be an import. It dates from around 1650–1550 BC.

NEW THEMES

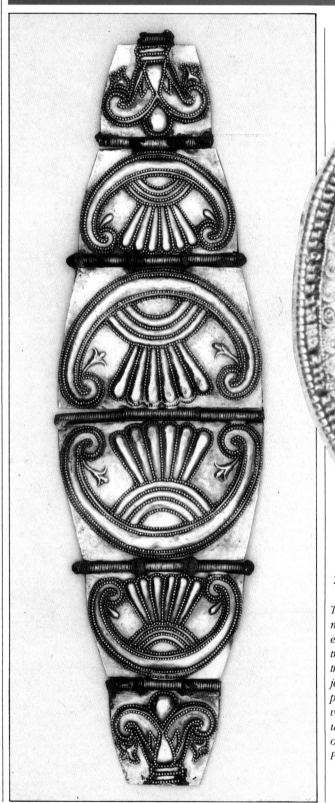

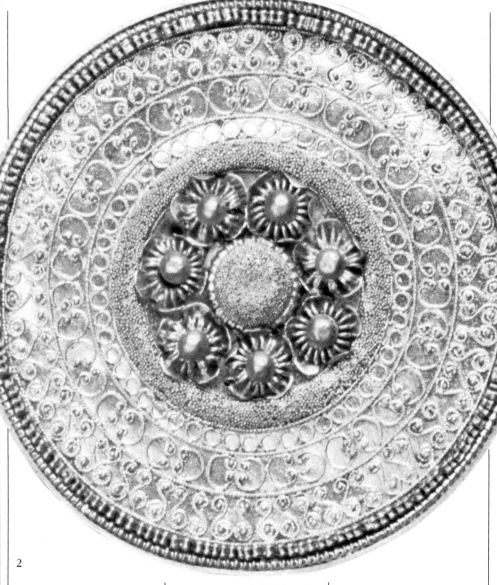

2

The early centuries of the first millennium BC saw the establishment of Phoenician traders and colonists throughout the Mediterranean. Phoenician jewelry is characterized by its precise granulation work and its visually strong design. The motifs used were often Egyptian in origin, but the realization was Phoenician. The Phoenician bracelet (**1**) looks almost Art Deco whereas the repeated motif might derive from the Egyptian hieroglyph for "gold." The bracelet is from Sardinia and dates from the 7th-6th centuries BC.

The precision of even Phoenician goldwork was surpassed by the Etruscans, in central Italy. The highly intricate, if not overcrowded, disk earring (**2**) is of about the same age as the Phoenician bracelet, but the granulation and filigree are on a much smaller scale. Etruscan techniques and assembly methods, however, were based on Phoenician ones. For example, the corroded hinge pinss of the Phoenician bracelet are of silver – a metal used for similar structural purposes in Etruscan goldwork.

1

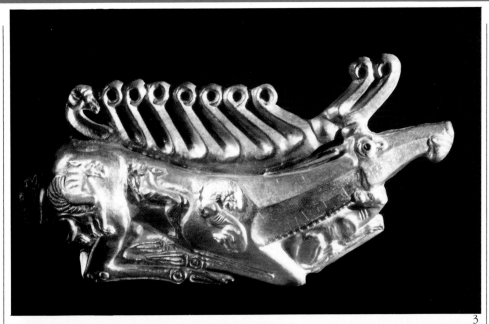

3

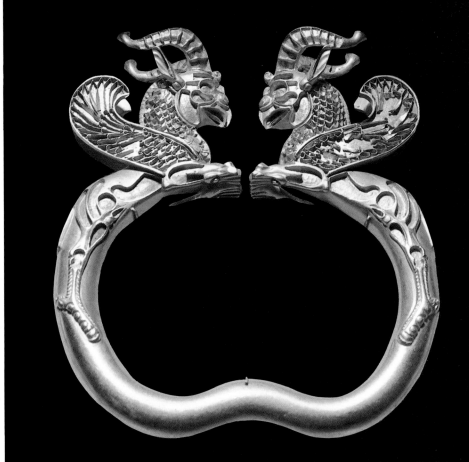

5

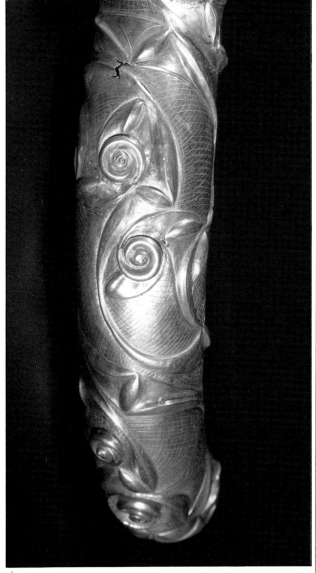

4

The naturalistic jewelry styles that spread through the Middle East and Europe in the first millennium BC probably derived from the Russian steppes, the home of the gold stag (3). This stag, probably a shield ornament, combines various animal forms and dates from around 500 BC.

Interactions with Persian and Greek forms resulted in a less barbaric animal style. The

magnificent armlet with griffin terminals (5), one of a pair from the so-called Oxus Treasure, dates from around 400 BC. It was originally all inlaid with stones.

The naturalistic designs of Celtic Europe can have for us an Art Nouveau appearance, as in the detail of a gold torque of the 1st century BC, from Broighter, in Ireland (4).

AFTER ALEXANDER

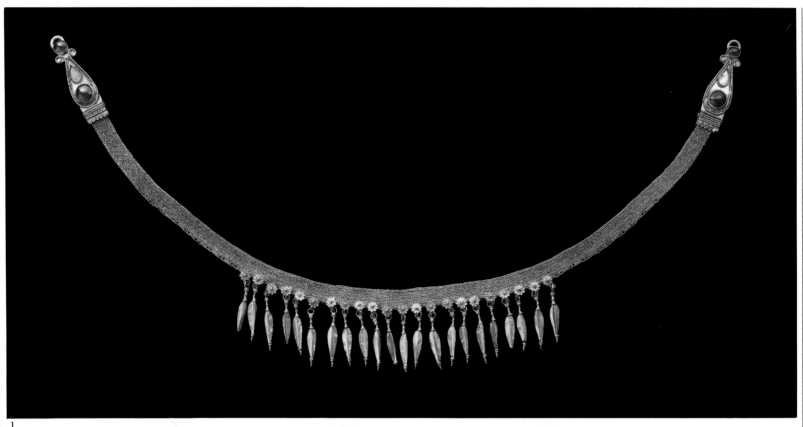

1

The necklace shown above (**1**) dates to around 300 BC and is of a type popular in the Hellenistic world, established by the conquests of Alexander the Great. A strap-like band of several narrow chains joined side by side supports a fringe of small spearhead and rosette pendants. The terminals are enlivened with garnets. Necklets of this type were worn suspended by pins from shoulder to shoulder rather than around the neck.

Hellenistic jewelry was often decorated with enamel, usually blue and green, but much of this has decayed with time. The enamel was normally positioned in cells formed from wire. This is the case on the terminals flanking the gold and garnet Herakles knot centerpiece (**2**) of the 3rd century BC. The birds pendants on the earrings (**3**) consist of a gold framework dipped into white enamel. This dipped enamel technique seems to have been an Italian specialty of the 2nd to 1st **centuries** BC.

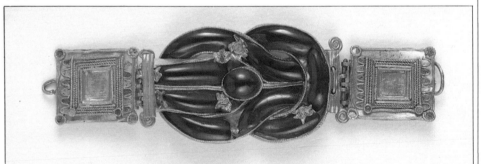

2

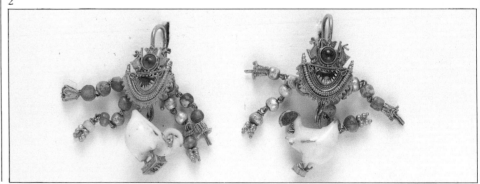

3

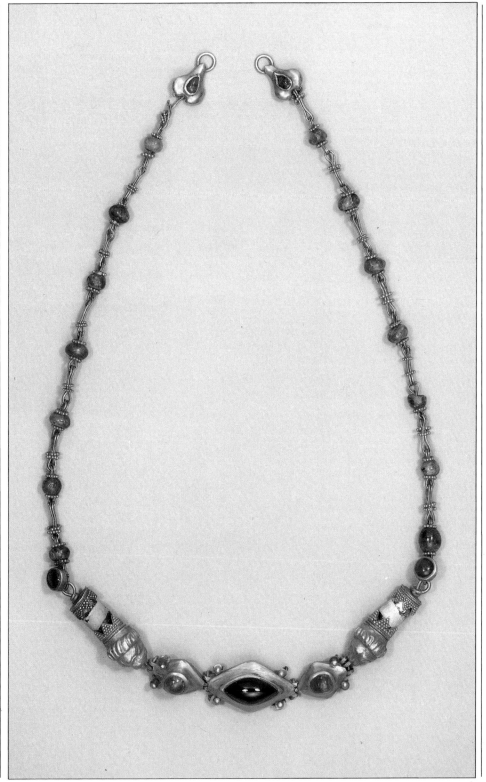

Jewelry from the Hellenistic period shows a growing love of colored stones and a trend away from elaborate filigree. The earring or pendant (**5**) and the necklet (**4**) show these changes in taste. The earring, a superb version of the well-known disk and lunate type, was found in southern Russia and dates to the end of the 4th century BC. The decoration consists of fine applied filigree work, and the only color is provided by the enamel placed in the filigree cells. The necklet consists of gold wire links threaded through emerald beads. This type of stone and gold linking is typical of the second half of the Hellenistic period. The lion-head terminals have banded black and white glass collars, and the centerpieces are set with emeralds and a garnet. This necklet, from Asia Minor, dates from c. 150–50 BC.

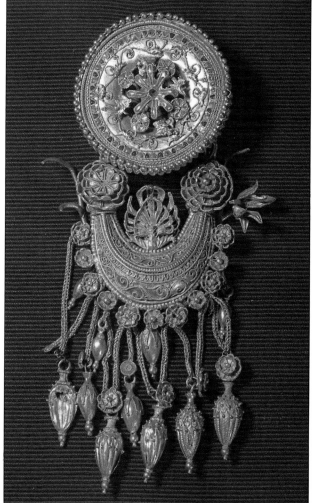

4

5

PAGANS AND CHRISTIANS

The elaborate gold collar, of which a detail is shown here (1), comes from Sweden and dates from the 6th century AD. Nevertheless the technical and stylistic approach shown in the granulation and filigree links back through three millennia to the Mediterranean and Middle East.

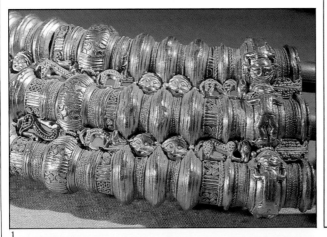

1

CONTRACTS

In the Roman period, as in earlier times, the evidence we have for the day-to-day trade of the goldsmith comes from pictorial and textual evidence. It seems possible that the introduction of precious metal coinage by about 600 BC helped the jeweler by providing a ready means by which the man in the street could obtain gold. Certainly in the Hellenistic and Roman periods there is far more evidence regarding the purchase of jewelry by ordinary people.

The dry sands of Egypt have allowed the survival of a vast number of papyrus documents which

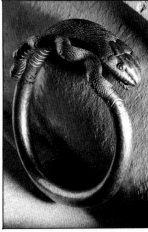

A gold armlet in the form of a smake of the 1st century AD, probably from Egypt.

shed light on all aspects of life in Egypt in the Roman period. Among these documents are several dealing with jewelry transactions. One of these relates to an order for a pair of gold coiled snake armlets to be made for a customer. The document records that money was given by the customer with which the goldsmith was to purchase the gold. Snake armlets of the type that the document is probably referring to can be seen worn in pairs on the upper arms of women in 1st-century AD funerary depictions, as here on the gilded mummy mask

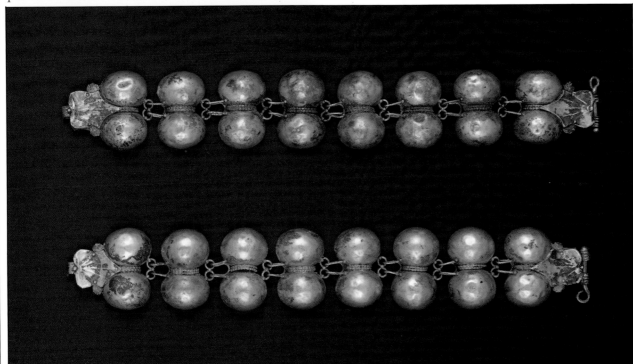

Goldwork from Pompeii and the neighboring towns destroyed by the eruption of Vesuvius in 79 AD reveals a rather stark geometric style. The dome bracelets (2) are a characteristic example.

Close links can be seen between some jewelry from Pompeii and that of the same period from Egypt. The magnificent gilded mummy covering (3) depicts snake armlets (as above), snake bracelets (maybe a funerary convention and not an everyday style), earrings, necklets, and rings. The latter include a snake ring on the third finger of the right hand, the normal finger for such rings.

2

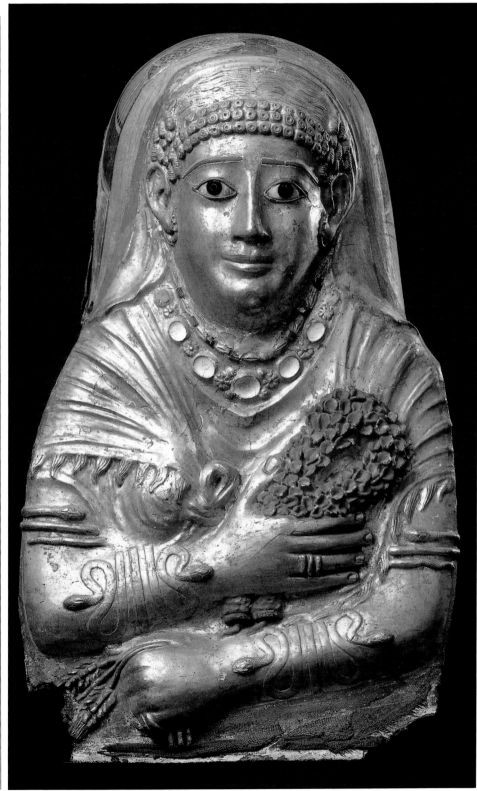

3

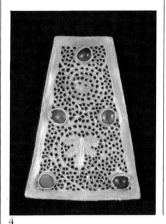

4

Both dome bracelets and the gilt mask date to the 1st century AD.

The more Hellenistic tastes of the eastern Roman and early Byzantine periods contrast with the plainer Pompeian and early Romano-Egyptian styles.

A fine chisel-pierced openwork technique, as seen in the 4th-century AD necklet element from Asia Minor (4), was most popular in the early Byzantine period. (This gold and garnet element was stolen in 1982 and has not been recovered.)

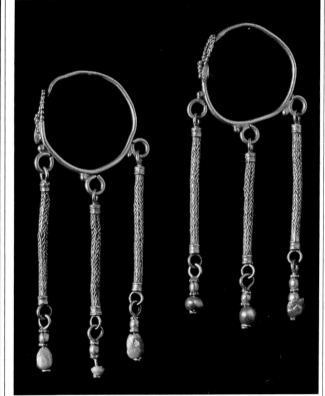

5

The hoop earrings, with their finely linked chain drops and pearls (5), are a good example of the simpler designs of some Byzantine jewelry. These probably come from Egypt and can be dated to the 5th to 6th centuries AD. The small gold granules where the pendant rings join the hoops help strengthen the joint and are typical of the type.

THE DARK AGES

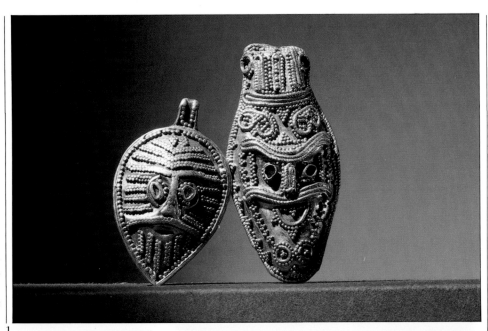

The goldwork of the so-called Dark Ages can be compared favorably with anything produced before or since. This is as true of technique as it is of style and design. This can be illustrated by taking, as an example, the jewelry produced by the Vikings.

The two pendants in the form of faces (**1**), of silver not gold, date from around 800–1000 AD. In technique they are most visually reminiscent of Phoenician work (particularly that from Spain) –

though the Phoenicians seemingly could not produce granulation in silver.

The gold strap end (**3**) also shows fine quality filigree and granulation work. This dates from about the 9th-century AD and was found in Norway.

The gold disk (**2**) from Sweden is the largest Viking example of a type of pendant termed a bracteate. The center shows a stylized human head and a horse and is based on a coin.

1

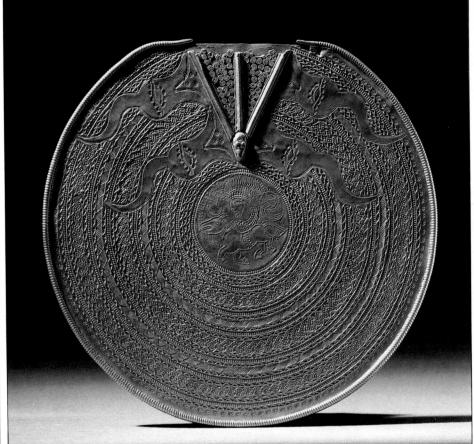

2

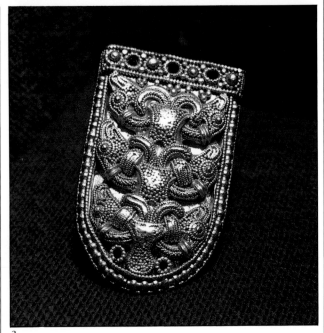

3

One of the characteristics of Post-Roman European jewelry is the use of cloisonné set stones, most usually thin, flat slivers of garnet. These can be seen in a

7th-century belt buckle from Aker, in Norway (**4**), plated with gold and silver and decorated with niello work.

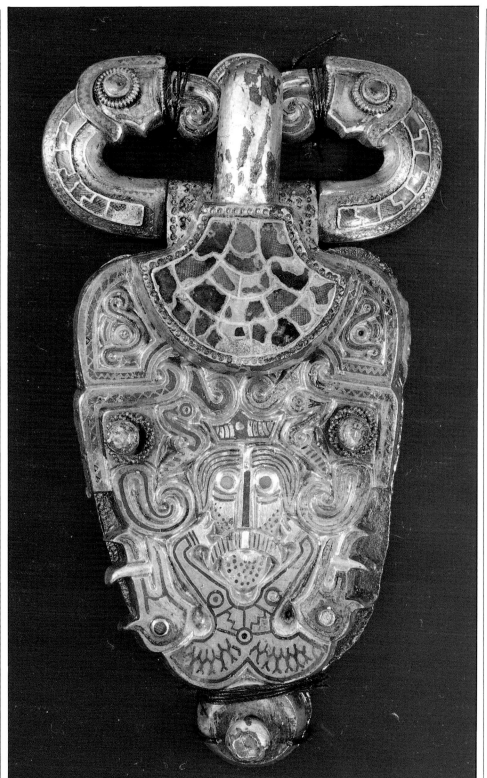

4

Animal motifs, less obvious in the buckle, are clearly seen in the silver bracelet from Sweden of the 11th century (**5**). The plaited hoop is typical Viking.

Ring brooches were popular in the Roman period and typical of Medieval jewelry. The two Viking Period examples (**6**) act as a perfect link between the ancient and medieval goldsmith's craft.

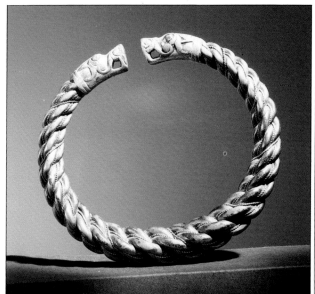

5

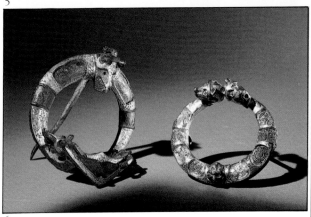

6

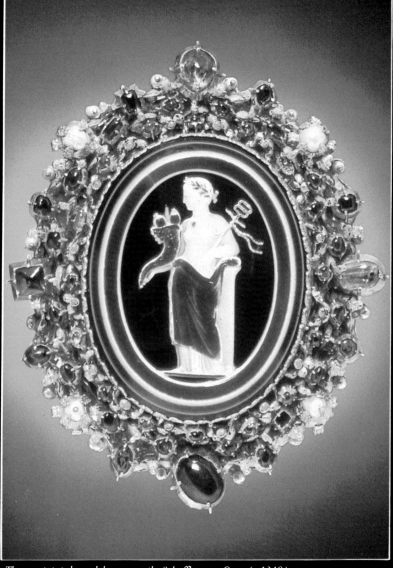

The great state brooch known as the Schaffhausen Onyx (c.1240).

CHAPTER TWO

THE MEDIEVAL CRAFTSMEN

800-1500

The Middle Ages

·

The Byzantine legacy

·

Gothic influences

RONALD LIGHTBOWN

INTRODUCTION

The early Middle Ages – the period from AD 800, when Charlemagne was crowned emperor of the West, to about 1200 – saw the gradual emergence of a distinct European culture out of the confusion of the so-called Dark Ages. With the relative political and economic stability that had been achieved by the 12th century came a wonderful renaissance of artistic and intellectual life, born of the clash of two traditions – the classical tradition and the tradition of native art which had persisted throughout the long centuries of wars and migrations.

The artistic achievements of the Teutonic tribes who

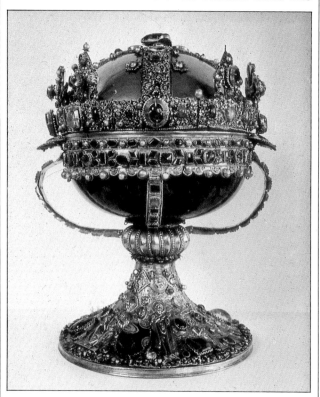

swept through Europe remind us that although they might have been barbarians, these people were also capable of producing some of the most beautiful metalwork ever known, whose intricate and mysterious designs appear to us all the more extraordinary because so little is known of the people who created them.

From the age of Charlemagne to around 1200 jewelry designs echoed those of imperial Byzantium. Byzantine art must have been the inspiration of the robes trimmed with broad borders sewn with pearls and stones, the earrings, the bracelets, the heavy collars, the jeweled girdles that we know to have been worn by great men and women in Carolingian and Ottonian times – although not all jewelry worn was as Byzantine as the great gold parure of an imperial lady, dating from about 1000, which was formerly

known as the treasure of the Empress Gisela (see page 39). Here the pectoral ornament is wholly Byzantine in style, with its gems strung on long thin wires so that they glittered on the breast like drops of color. The earrings are of the crescent form popular in the early Middle Ages and are also Byzantine in origin, and the brooch is domed and composed of concentric circles, again probably a Byzantine design. Such great brooches, in their stately richness were typical of the majestic jewelry of the early Middle Ages, where the effect sought was one of heavy jeweled splendor produced by the combination of monumentality of form with intricacy of surface decoration, often created by scrolls of filigree sometimes inset with small stones.

The Use of Stones

In the early Middle Ages a greater range of stones was employed in jewelry than was the custom from the beginning of the 13th century. As well as the four great precious stones of the Middle Ages, the sapphire, the ruby, the emerald, and the diamond, turquoises and topazes were used, again suggesting Byzantine influence and a taste for a wide variety of color. We do not know when this taste disappeared, but certainly from about 1200 jewels of gold were principally set with sapphires, rubies, emeralds, and diamonds, with pearls in their pure, milky opalescence used for contrast. Of these stones the most highly prized were the sapphire and the ruby, the sapphire being perhaps the more greatly valued up to the 14th century, when the ruby rose into high favor. True rubies were comparatively rare; far commoner was the spinel ruby, known in the Middle Ages as the balas ruby after its place of origin, Badakshan, in northeastern Afghanistan.

Although there may have been some limited knowledge of how to cut or shape these stones, before the 14th century they were usually simply polished, so that most early medieval stones are cabochon stones, and keep something of the irregularity of their natural form. The art of cutting and faceting stones became much commoner during the 14th century, and during the latter 1300s the art of cutting the diamond was mastered for the first time. At first the cuts were naturally not very elaborate: sapphires and rubies could be cut into eight facets, diamonds into points, and all stones could be table-cut. There is evidence to suggest that much more elaborate cutting and faceting began in the 15th century in the Netherlands, which have since remained the great center of stone cutting, though the rise of Amsterdam as the capital of the art belongs to a much later period.

Jewels were made in the Middle Ages by goldsmiths, rather than by specialist jewelers, who begin to appear only in the late 14th century. Stones were either set in collets or mounted in claw settings *à jour,* a technique that allows light to be reflected through the stone. Stones were tinctured or foiled to improve their color, and this could and did lead to malpractices that called forth much legislation from the early 13th century onward. In general, medieval regulations, though seriously concerned with purity and genuineness of metal, reveal less anxiety about the silver and gold used in jewels, since their quantity was small, than about the stones. It was usually forbidden to set gold with semiprecious stones, such as amethysts or garnets which were cheaper alternatives for true precious stones, or with the substitute stones of glass and crystal, often tinctured doublets, which were much produced from early times and later became a specialty of Paris. In the cheaper metal silver, on the other hand, it was forbidden to use genuine precious stones. It is plain both from documents and surviving jewels that fraud and deception were extensively practiced in the Middle Ages, and that it behooved the purchaser of jewels and precious stones to be on his guard. Sometimes no doubt mistakes were genuine, for gemology was not yet a very advanced science.

Major Centers and Techniques

The centers for the making of jewelry in the Middle Ages were the great cities of Paris, Cologne, and Venice, with Paris enjoying the supremacy in fashion from about 1200 to 1400 that it was to regain in the 18th and 19th centuries. As goldsmith's work medieval jewelry represents the major goldsmiths' styles of the Middle Ages in miniature: thus 11th- and 12th-century jewelry has the characteristics of Ottonian and Romanesque goldsmiths' work, which in turn reflects the major design styles of its age. The main decorative technique of medieval jewelry was enameling, in its successive forms: cloisonné enamel derived from Byzantium; *champlevé* enamel; translucent enamel, introduced about 1290; and *émail en ronde bosse,* introduced or revived about 1360. Another source of ornament, used in brooches, was the cameo. Antique cameos were as highly prized and eagerly collected in the Middle Ages as they were in the Renaissance, though not with the same spirit of reverence for the art of antiquity. Brooches such as the Schaffhausen Onyx of *c.* 1330–40 show how richly and magnificently such cameos were mounted to make state brooches. Such a brooch would certainly be worn only on great occasions; according to the documents, the best jewelry was for high and holiday wear, and the second-best for more ordinary occasions.

The 13th century, a period of great self-confidence in Western European art, saw notable changes in the style and types of jewelry that were worn. Jewelry seems to have become much lighter in spirit under the influence of the Gothic style, which was first evident in jewelry in the second quarter of the 13th century in Paris, and gradually influenced the style of jewelry elsewhere in Western Europe. For the heavy, rounded forms of earlier jewels it

This fleur de lis brooch of silver-gilt, probably for a mantle, is decorated with champlevé *enamel and set with stones which are among the earliest cut stones known from the Middle Ages. It dates from the early 14th century. The* fleur-de-lys *was the official badge of the French royal house, and the brooch was preserved among the French royal regalia at the Abbey of Saint-Denis.*

substituted angular or lobed designs; it replaced their three-dimensional richness with lighter, flatter, two-dimensional designs, in which stones and pearls are isolated against the metal. At the same time earrings and bracelets disappear, except in southern Italy and Sicily, where lingering Byzantine influence, and, in Spain, Moorish influence, kept them in fashion until the end of the Middle Ages. On the heads of noble men and women appears the coronal, or crown, whose distinguishing mark was its fleurons. Lighter and less solemn head ornaments were the chaplet and garland, much worn by wealthy bourgeois men and women as well as by their superiors in degree. Women's hair was bound and wound into tresses and other forms by bands known as *tressoirs,* which were often jeweled, sometimes very richly. At the neck was worn a brooch, which might be a simple ring-brooch, at its plainest a plain utilitarian fastener, or a great cluster brooch formed around a cameo. The heavy collars of earlier times disappeared and were replaced by light chains or laces or ribands from which hung pendants, either inside or outside the dress.

Such pendants were often worn to give protection to the wearer. They could take the form of a sacred symbol like a cross, or of a container for holy relics, or of single stones, which were believed to have certain virtues. To all precious and semiprecious stones were assigned special virtues of protection or power. If they were worn as ligatures or suspensions – that is, either clasping the arm or finger in the form of riband bracelets or rings, or hung round the neck – their virture would affect the wearer. Clerics and nuns, for instance, wore sapphires because the sapphire was believed to encourage chastity and chill lust; similary the ruby, a stone of lordly fieriness, was worn by princes. There was also a belief in the protective force of magical formula and characters – inscribed on brooches we find inscriptions that are a jumble of letters whose meaning was always secret; familar words of power such as *abracadabra*, others less familar like *ananizupta;* phrases from the Gospels which were believed to have special virtue, and invocations of Mary, the Three Magi, and the saints.

Pendants later developed into cluster or cameo forms, often in imitation of brooches, which were the commonest jewels of the Middle Ages. The brooch itself, at the beginning of the 13th century, was still usually either a cluster or a cameo. But we also find figurative motifs. These were sometimes symbolic, like the lion or the eagle, both longstanding symbols of princely power - the eagle appears in rich brooches in the 11th century. Then by about 1300 we begin to find lighter motifs intended to amuse or delight the eye – a parrot, an elephant, or butterfly.

Around the waist of the rich and noble was worn a girdle, with a buckle and tag (pendant) of silver or gold. The girdle might be decorated with enamel, or set with precious stones, or, more often, embroidered with pearls. Form the late 13th century we even hear of girdles made wholly of links of silver or gold, but massive girdles of this type were never common, even in the 14th century when they sometimes took the form of chains. Those who were either rich and ostentatious or noble also fastened their mantles with cloak clasps in precious metal which either linked together or held ornamental cords or straps.

Enamel Ornament

In the 14th century, with the triumph of the Gothic style in architecture, architectural forms are introduced into jewelry, and niches, canopies, and crockets begin to ornament even humbler articles such as girdle buckles and cloak clasps. The whole spirit is one of elegance and grace rather than stateliness and loaded richness. We now find lovers on brooches, jewels in the form of letters or decorated with little scenes in enamel. Then toward the end of the 14th century wholly new fashions appear in jewelry, originating once more in Paris. The technique of *émail en ronde bosse,* in which enamel – usually white with colored details – is applied to sculptural motifs executed in gold, became popular from the late 1360s and seems to have introduced a whole new vocabulary of naturalistic and romantic motifs into jewelry and especially into brooches. Prominent among these was a white lady, sometimes sitting under a pavilion in a garden; there were brooches of flowers and trees – a white rose, violets, hawthorn; of birds and animals – a lark, a partridge, a pheasant, a doe, a white hart lying under a white flower, a white flower with two squirrels, a falcon, a maiden, and a unicorn; of noble ladies, perhaps seated in a sunburst, as in one brooch, as in one brooch, or standing among white flowers and holding a parrot as in another. There was also a vogue for jewelry figuring or decorated with chivalric devices – the symbols adopted by princes and great men as their own special badges. The white hart, assumed as a device by Richard II about 1390, for instance, was worn as a badge or brooch by his retainers and also by his kinsfolk, such as the Duchess of Burgundy. Jewels of this style, in their pure bright color and elegance of motif, are among the most beautiful of the later Middle Ages.

Cluster and cameo brooches nevertheless still remained popular, and in the early 15th century there emerged a new taste for jewelry setting off single stones or simply composed of stones in juxtaposition. This fashion was related to developments in the art of stone cutting. The metal now provided at most a frame, and might only be a mere setting for the stones. A favorite setting for a single stone was at the center of an enameled flower, usually a rose, or in a flower on a stem. The wealthy dukes of Burgundy had a jewel of this kind known as the White Rose Jewel. One of the most famous 15th-century jewels, composed of juxtaposed stones, was also theirs: the famous Three Brothers Brooch captured by the Swiss from Charles the Bold at Grandson in 1467.

Vogues for luxury in dress and jewelry swept the Middle Ages at various times, notably in the later 13th and early 14th centuries and again in the late 14th century. They led to a preoccupation with the unusual and the fantastic in the cut, color, and shape of dress, and to the transformation into jewels or ornaments of anything that could be treated in this way. Clerics might thunder from pulpits and magistrates try to check extravagance, but buttons of silver, of amber, of mother-of-pearl; spangles of beaten gold or silver; rich embroidery of pearls; and braids of gold decorated with pearls and precious stones all shone and glittered on the fine man and lady of the later Middle Ages. The bracelet reappeared in the 1390s, and became a chivalric love token, while the collar re-emerged from the 1380s to hang once more either closely around a lady's neck or loosely over her shoulders. Men also might wear collars, and massive chains of gold or silver or silver-gilt glittered on the breasts of knights and noblemen these fashions inspired by a desire to demonstrate the prestige associated with belonging to one of the orders of knighthood.

Medieval jewelry, with its unfaceted or boldly shaped stones, is perhaps the most poetical in range of feeling of

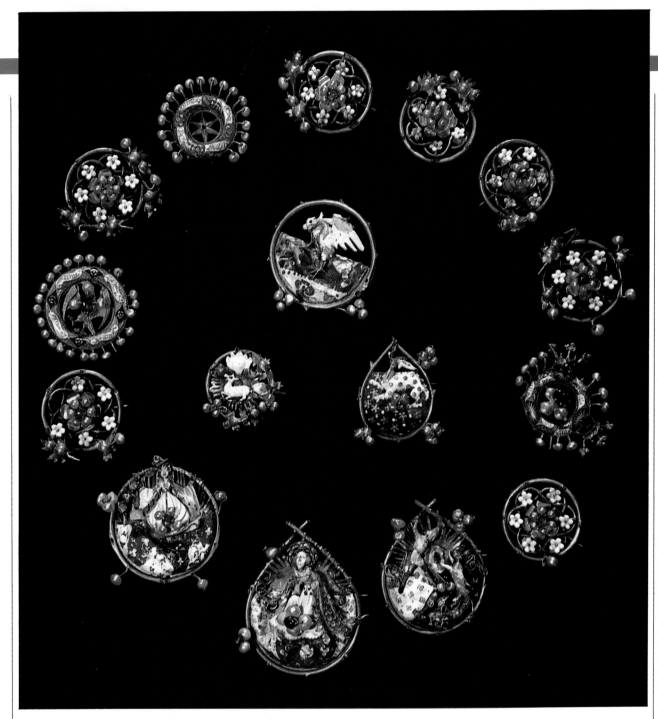

The Essen brooches, which may originate from a collar, are of gold, delicately enameled in the technique of émail en ronde bosse. *They show the range of fanciful and lively naturalistic motifs that became popular in brooches from the late 14th century – a white lady, flowers, a swan, a huntsman with dog and hare, a kid. They were probably made at Cologne, c. 1400-20.*

any jewelry ever made. It can be mystical, romantic, playful: it can suggest the mysteries of heaven, or the amorous delights of the lover's garden, or the nobility and prestige of knighthood. Perhaps it is the purity of the colors and the glow of the metal that are the final secrets of its delicate power.

INFLUENCES

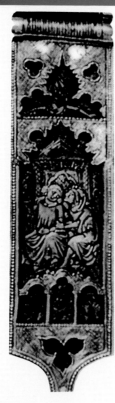

1

This Italian 14th century girdle (**1**) of silver parcel gilt and decorated with translucent enamel, shows how the forms of Gothic architecture, as demonstrated in this detail (**2**) of the west façade of Salisbury cathedral (1220-58), were borrowed by goldsmiths and developed into a miniature ornamental vocabulary for jewelry. When applied to the mounts of a girdle (detail), the style has a fantastic appearance which probably pleased patrons of the 14th century, who sought gaiety and strangeness in all they wore.

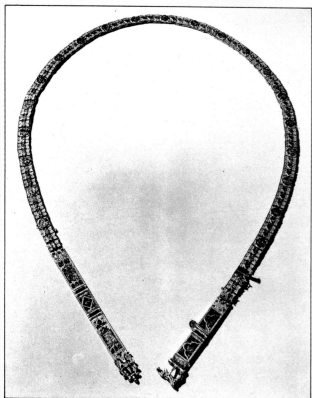

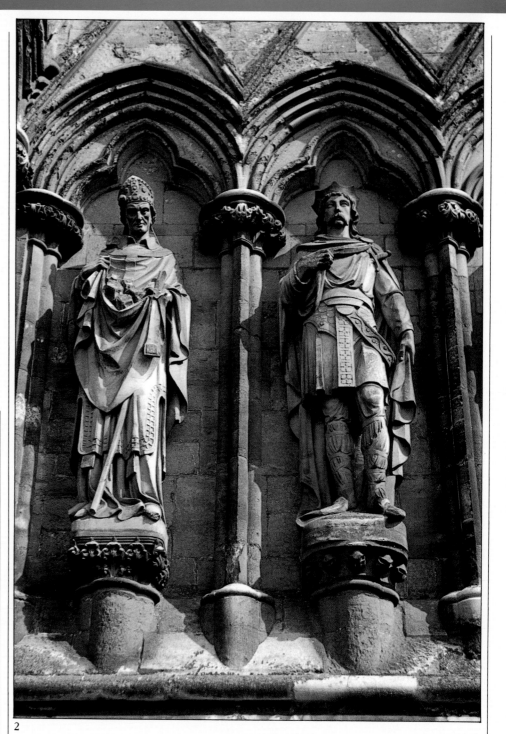

2

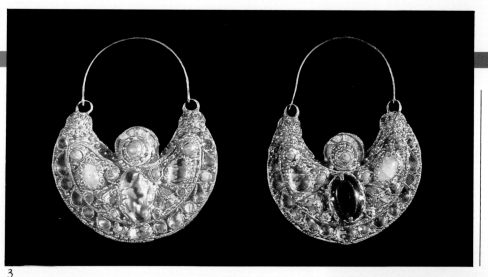

Set with stones and pearls, these gold earrings of c. 1000, from the Gisela Treasure (3), show the influence of Byzantine jewelry on Imperial German court jewelry. The crescent shape was borrowed from Byzantium, whose imperial dress and jewelry set the fashion for the Emperors of the West.

3

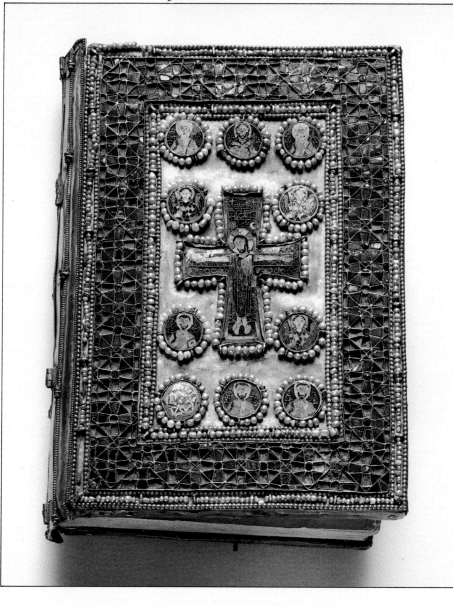

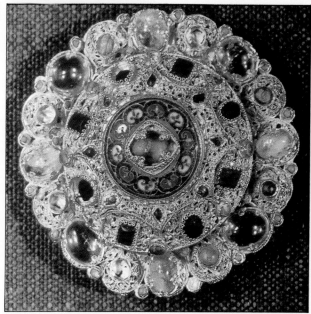

4

This circular domed brooch of c. 1000 (4), also from the Gisela Treasure, is again probably inspired by Byzantine jewelry. It is of gold, set with stones and pearls, and with a ring of cloisonné enamel around the central sapphire. The effect is monumental, but with a barbaric glow of color. A 9th-century

Byzantine book cover (5) set with pearls shows the sort of precious Byzantine enamels on gold that were so much admired in the early medieval West. They are executed in the technique of cloisonné, in which the enamel colors are separated by fine walls of gold.

5

EARLY GOLD AND ENAMEL WORK

(1) *This gold and enamel eagle brooch of c. 1000 is part of a treasure of jewels found at Mainz in 1886 which must have belonged to an imperial German lady and was once associated with the* *Empress Gisela (d. 1026). The eagle was a symbol at this period of imperial rule; here it is copied from Byzantium.*

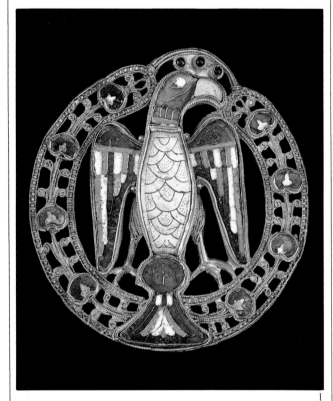

1

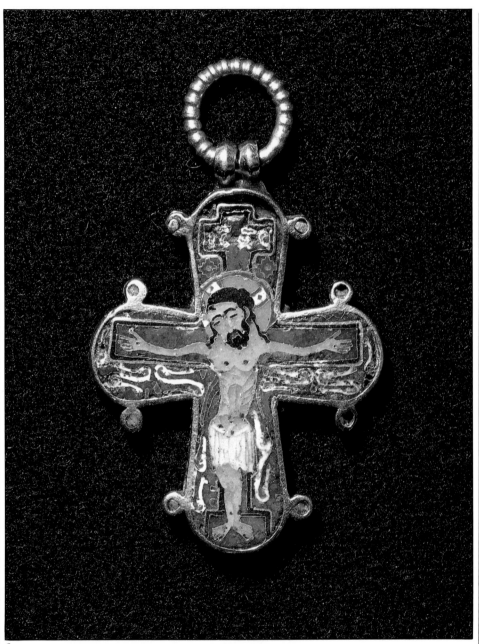

2

Medieval people frequently wore small pendant crosses of this kind, hung from a lace or chain. This cross (2), c. 1000, is known as the Dagmar Cross. Made of gold and *decorated with cloisonné enamel, it was found in the grave of Queen Dagmar of Denmark (d. 1212). It may have come from Byzantium or from south Italy. We are not* *sure how it reached Denmark, but Byzantine crosses and other ornaments were very popular in Scandinavia.*

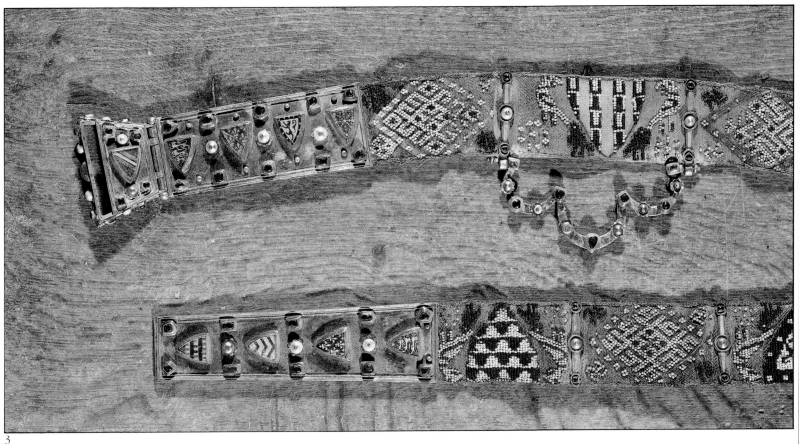

3

This rich girdle of c. 1270 was found on the body of the Infante Fernando de la Cerda (d.1275) son of King Alfonso the Wise of Castile, when his tomb in Las Huelgas, Burgos, was opened (3). The coats-of-arms suggest that it is really English, and was a gift to him, perhaps from Edmund of Lancaster, a son of Henry III. The hoop is for suspending a purse.

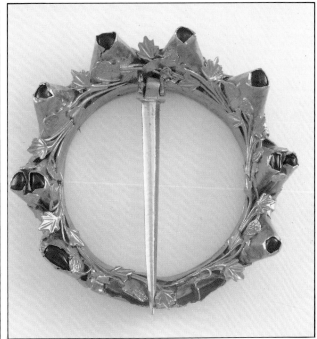

4

Ring-brooches were often plain or simply decorated, but they could also be treated as richly showy ornaments. This beautiful late 13th-century example (4) is of gold, set with sapphires and rubies, with vine leaf scrolls between the collets. It is probably French.

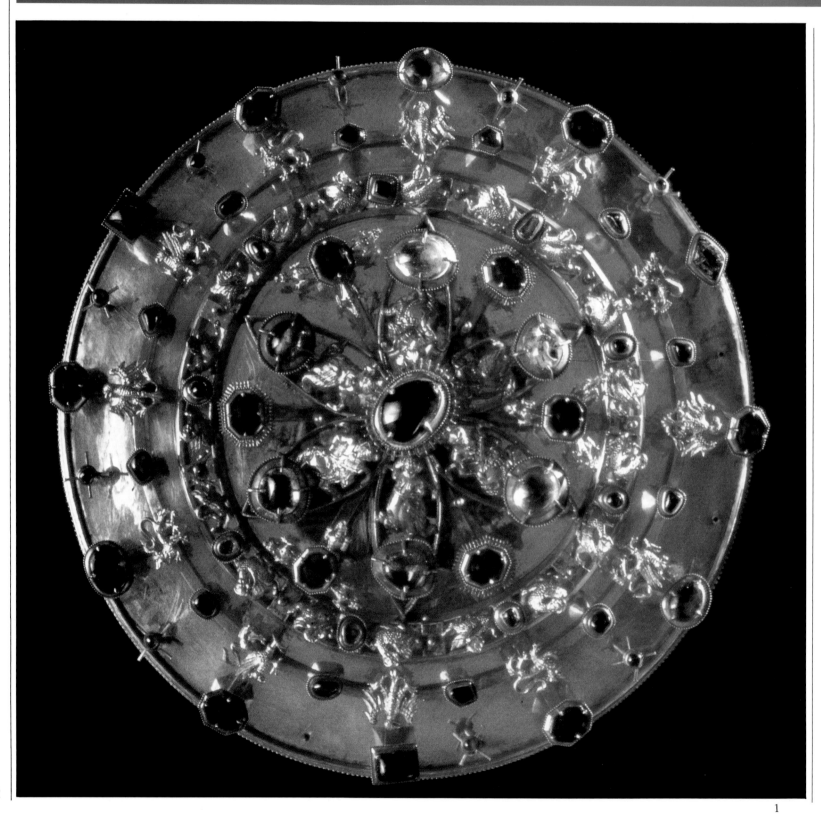

1

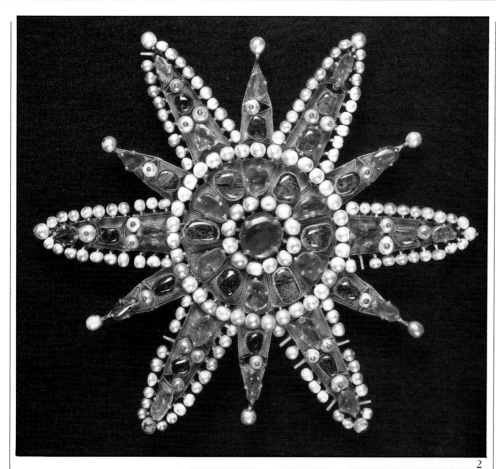

2

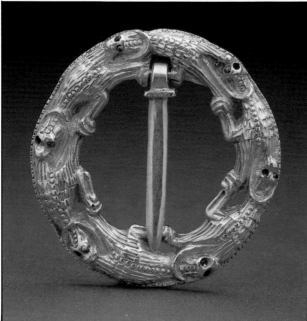

4

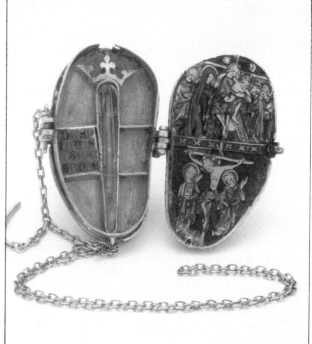

3

Patterned in dazzling red and green with amethysts and emeralds, and with pearls, this great gold star brooch (*2*) is one of the most beautiful of 14th-century jewels. It was probably made in Venice or Verona about 1350 for a lady of the Della Scala family, lords of Verona, the city where it was discovered in 1939. It shows the large, bold forms of rich Italian jewelry in the mid-14th century and was probably worn on the upper part of a robe. The Pendant of the Holy Thorn (*3*) is a royal French jewel, c. 1320-30, designed to contain a relic of a thorn from the Crown of Thorns, bought by St Louis from the Emperor of Constantinople. It consists of two foiled crystals, mounted in silver-gilt and hinged to a center case. They open to show scenes in translucent enamel. The case contains the Holy Thorn itself.

The place where this gold brooch was made is a mystery, but it was probably the work of a German or French goldsmith working for a Scandinavian king or queen (*1*). It was found in the Motala river in Sweden in the early 14th century. The ethereal colors of the stones – rubies, sapphires, emeralds, and pearls – are relieved by figures and monsters.

The gold Kames brooch of c. 1300 shows another method of enriching the form of a ring-brooch, for it is designed as a round of dragons, with eyes of yellow glass, biting each other's tails (*4*). The back has an inscription of the names of Jesus, the Three Magi, and the Fate Atropa, all believed to protect the wearer from various kinds of harm.

CEREMONIAL JEWELS

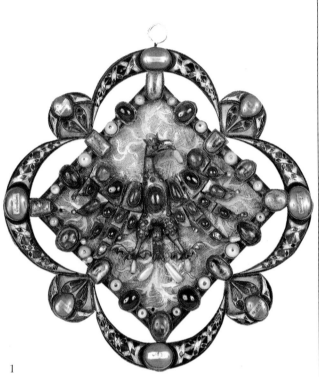

1

This reliquary pendant of silver-gilt, set with emeralds, sapphires, rubies, and crystals (*1*), was probably made in Bohemia c. 1350-70. Under the stones in the lobes are small relics. The engraved flames behind may be the device of St Wenceslas of Bohemia.

(*2*) The Wilton Diptych, painted c. 1395, shows Richard II of England wearing a collar of broom-cod, the device of Charles VI of France, and his own device of a white hart, which he assumed in 1390. Badges of this kind were given in the late 14th and 15th centuries by kings and princes to their intimate household knights and to their relatives, friends, and supporters. Richard was accused by his opponents of trying to create a faction by his gifts of hart-badges.

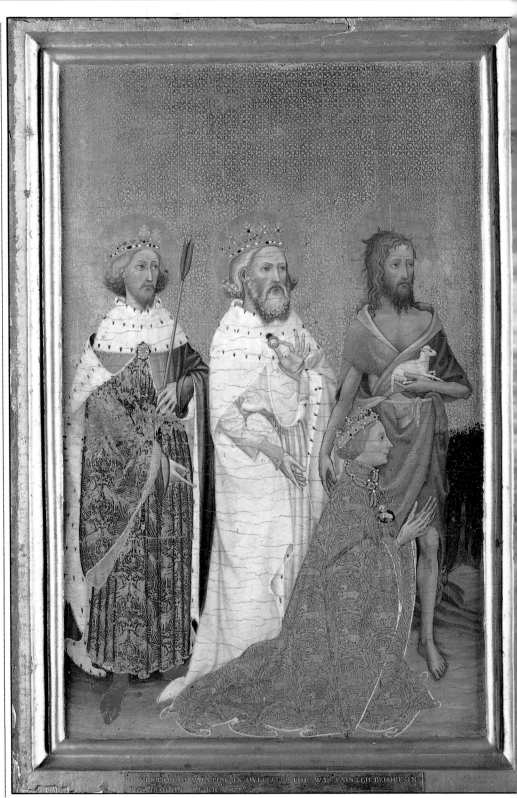

2

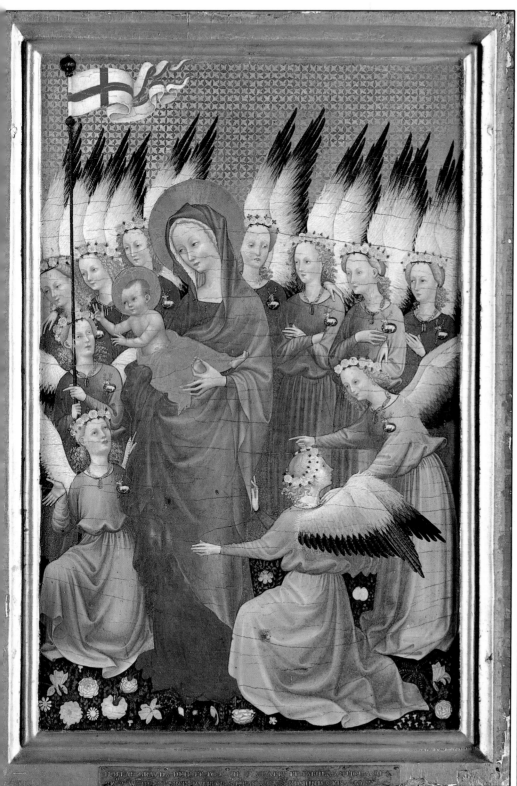

Princess Blanche, daughter of Henry IV, took this English royal crown to Bavaria on her marriage (3). It is of gold, set with rubies, sapphires, diamonds, and pearls. The high, spiring pinnacles are typical of late 14th-century crowns; this one was made either in France or, more probably, *England. The two cloak-clasps (4) of silver gilt and enamel were made for King Louis the Great of Hungary and given by him to his chapel in Aachen in about 1374. They show the heraldic magnificence of such ornaments, worn only by the noblest in the land.*

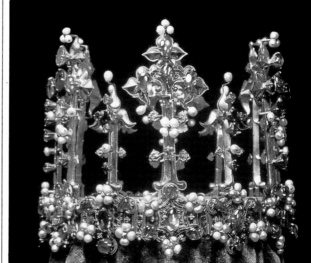

3

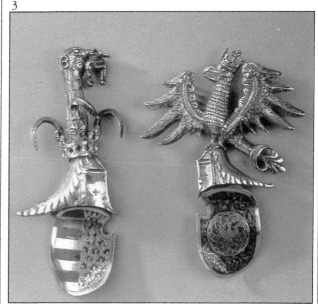

4

FIGURATIVE WORK

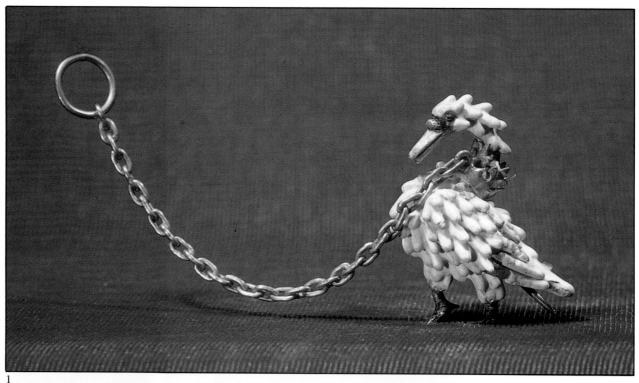

1

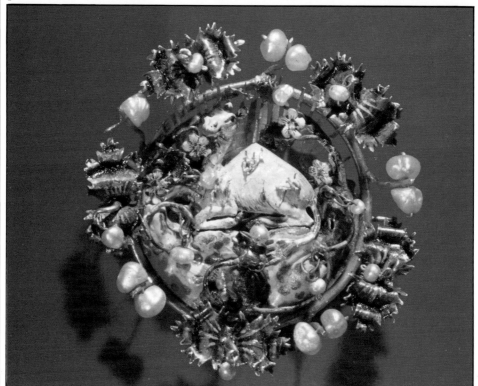

2

The Swan Jewel, from the first half of the 15th century, is of gold, enameled in the technique of émail en ronde bosse (1). It was found in Dunstable, England. The crown around its neck suggests that it may have been a royal badge, but it may equally have belonged to someone from one of the great English families claiming descent from the Swan Knight. A love of the exotic, one of the leading tastes of fashionable people in the late 14th and early 15th centuries is exemplified in this dromedary brooch. Of gold, enameled white and green, it combines intricacy of surface with poetry of feeling and subtlety of workmanship (2).

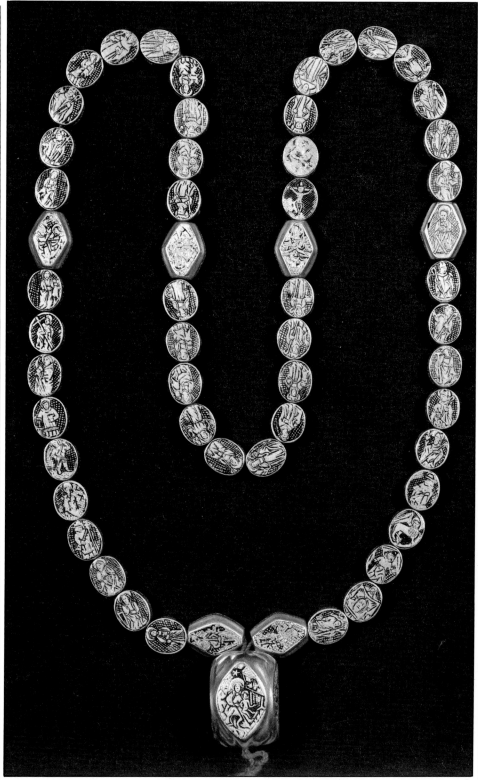

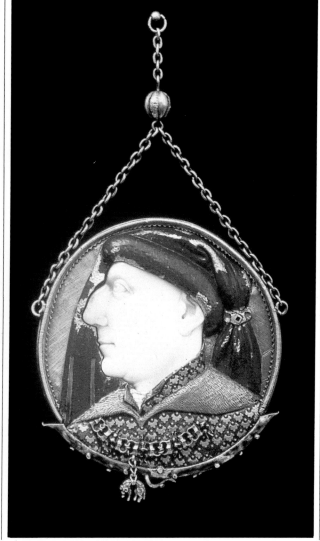

The Langdale rosary (3), English, c. 1490-1500, is one of only two gold paternosters to survive from the Middle Ages. Its beads are enameled with the figures of saints, each carefully identified; the larger beads, known as "gauds," were for marking the number of prayers recited. This magnificent portrait pendant (c. 1440) of gold enameled in the clear red much favored by later medieval goldsmiths, is set with a hardstone profile of a knight of the Order of the Golden Fleece, probably Duke Philip the Good of Burgundy (4). Portrait pendants were rare in the Middle Ages, and were made almost exclusively for French or French-influenced princes and princesses.

3 4

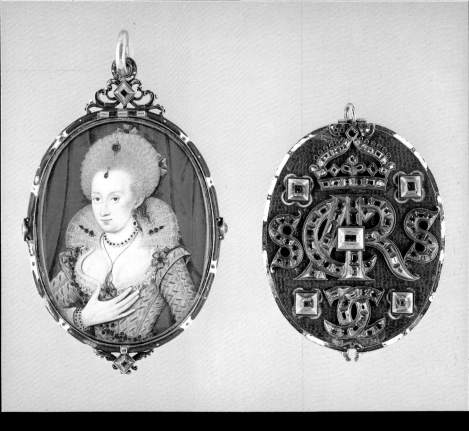

Nicholas Hilliard's exquisite miniature of Anne of Denmark, c. 1603 is contained in an enameled gold case with gold set diamonds, possibly from the workshop of George Heriot.

CHAPTER · THREE

RENAISSANCE AND BAROQUE JEWELS

1500-1714

Following fine art

·

Classicism

·

The French courts of the Bourbons

·

Death and politics

DIANA SCARISBRICK

INTRODUCTION

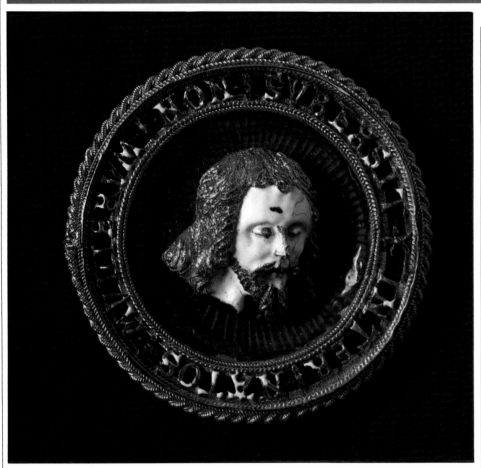

Jewelry in the Renaissance reached an artistic level comparable to that achieved in the fine arts. Artists as distinguished as Albrecht Dürer, Hans Holbein, and Giulio Romano were commissioned by princely patrons to produce designs that stimulated goldsmiths to bring their traditional skills of enameling, chasing, and casting to heights never since equaled. New motifs derived from classical art joined the medieval themes of religion and sentiment, which were re-interpreted.

The lead came from Italy, where the elegant but conservative designs of the 15th century were transformed into the exuberant and sculptural style associated with Benvenuto Cellini (1502–72). In his *Autobiography* Cellini recalls the fashion for hat badges in Rome at the outset of his career – successors to the medieval pilgrim and livery badges and, like them, worn in the upturned brim of the hat. Chased or embossed with scenes from the Bible, or from classical mythology or history, they declared cultural interests or spiritual aspirations. Modeled in gold, bright with enamels, and highlighted with colored gemstones and diamonds, they represent the fully evolved Renaissance style of jewelry. By the end of the 16th century this sculptural, elaborate style had given way to flatter, more decorative jewels in which stones play the principal role. An example of the latter is a heart-shaped hat jewel enclosing the ruby initials "DM" amid blue forget-me-nots which was found in the tomb of Count Otto Heinrich of Neuberg (1556–1604), at Lauingen on the Danube. His wife, Dorothea Maria, put it there..

Although the openwork style of the heart was new, the ornamental use of personal ciphers was not. Holbein's jewelry designs of the 1530s include a pendant with the initials "HI" for Henry VIII and Queen Jane Seymour, and "RE," perhaps for Enricus Rex. Mary Tudor owned a diamond necklace composed of "P"s and "M"s for herself and her husband, Philip II of Spain, and James I wore a hat badge with his wife's initial, "A" for Anne, likewise studded with diamonds. Holbein's historiated jewels carry longer inscriptions, and both necklaces and bracelets might be composed of letters spelling out messages in Latin or the vernacular, wrought in gold or studded with stones. The most prestigious of these monogram jewels were religious in character, representing the abbreviated Greek name of Christ, IHS, in Gothic or Roman capitals, and set with diamonds, the back enameled with the Instruments of Christ's Passion – crown of thorns, nails, scourge, and ladder. These were worn by Protestant men and women, who also wore crosses. Devotional jewelry reflecting Roman Catholic practices, especially veneration of the Virgin Mary, was restricted to those remaining loyal to the Papacy, particularly in Spain, where jeweled badges of the religious Confraternities and miniature representations of cult statues were a specialty.

Secular pendants pinned to the sleeve or hung from the neck demonstrate the diversity of Renaissance culture. They illustrate episodes from classical literature such as the stories of Diana and Actaeon, of Leda and the Swan, of Apollo and Daphne, of Cupid, busy firing his arrows at human hearts. Allegorical figures were popular: Charity with her children, Faith with her cross, Fortitude with her column; and in the last quarter of the 16th century they were contained in architectural settings in a style associated with the German designer Hans Collaert. The asymmetrical and distorted shapes of baroque pearls presented a particular challenge to the imagination, as well as to the technical skills of the Renaissance goldsmith, who transformed them into magnificent mermaids and tritons, warriors in armor, lions, rabbits, and wounded stags.

The Classical Influences

The classical revival, which provided the goldsmith with a vocabulary of divinities, nymphs, satyrs, heroes, pediments, and volutes, also brought with it a return to the difficult courtly art of gem engraving. Both intaglios – for signet rings – and cameos were set in Renaissance hat jewels, pendants, bracelets, and necklaces, in wrought-gold and jeweled frames. Some are reinterpretations of Roman themes – emperors and empresses, patriots and heroes – but others show an independent attitude to classical prototypes and are illustrations of events from the Bible or portraits of illustrious Renaissance men and women in contemporary dress. Rulers awarded their cameo portraits as a mark of the highest distinction: less rare, but almost as highly regarded, were miniatures in jeweled cases and medallic portraits, known as badges of honor, worn on long gold chains.

It was said that Sir Thomas Gresham, the founder of the Royal Exchange, invested his entire fortune in gold chains, and certainly every man and woman of standing wore them, in single or multiple rows and made of a variety of links, including knots imitating those in the ropes tied around the habits of Franciscan friars. Also worn at the neck were carcanets composed of richly chased and enameled gold links set with gemstones in high bezels, usually alternating with groups of milky-white pearls. Although narrower versions of these might be worn on the wrists, most bracelets were in the form of gold chains, individualized with ciphers, coats of arms and the betrothal symbols of hearts and hands on the clasps.

In the northern countries women's hair was covered with a French hood embellished with two rows of jewelry, known as biliments, and since the ears were covered, earrings were rare. But well before 1600 the French hood was out of fashion, and bodkins and aigrettes – like tufts of feathers – were pinned in hair padded out artificially and crowned with an "attire" of pearls strung into lace-like patterns on a wire frame. Besides earrings of pear pearls, there were others of goldsmith's work: ciphers, blackamoors, dolphins, and mermaids playing the lute.

Women's dresses, enriched by sets of buttons, were belted with jeweled bands matching carcanets, bracelets and biliments, or with rows of agate nuts sometimes enclosing figurative scenes. Hanging from the neck and girdle were useful items which the Renaissance goldsmith made into jewels: whistles designed as dragons, toothpicks like eagles' claws, fans with jeweled handles, furpieces with wrought-gold sable heads, and pomanders to scent the foul air.

Portraits show rings worn in profusion, and at no period have designs ever been so diverse. There are gimmel rings with double-hoop and twin bezels, symbolic of the married state, locket rings enclosing minute portraits, superb diamond rings made for royalty, signets engraved with complicated coats of arms, and each, notwithstanding the small scale, exemplifies the artistic spirit of the Renaissance.

The Rise of the Gemstone

In the 17th century this close connection with the fine arts came to an end as the craft of the jeweler was increasingly concerned with the display of stones rather than with the expression of intellectual con-

cepts, rank, occupation, religion, or political allegiance. From the reign of Henri IV and Marie de Medici, Paris was acknowledged as the center of taste and fashion. This ascendancy was confirmed by the splendor of Versailles under their grandson, Louis XIV. French designs were diffused abroad through pattern books, and the Revocation of the Edict of Nantes in 1685 drove so many Huguenot craftsmen out of France that in 1706 the Dowager Duchesse d'Orléans could observe that it was no longer true that pretty things had to be bought in Paris.

The supply of gemstones increased during the 17th century, but especially after the 1660s, when the East India Company gave the Marranos Portuguese Jews established in London permission to trade independently. At the same time the discovery of the laws of refraction and of the principles of analytical geometry stimulated progress in faceting and polishing. The rose cut with multiple facets had

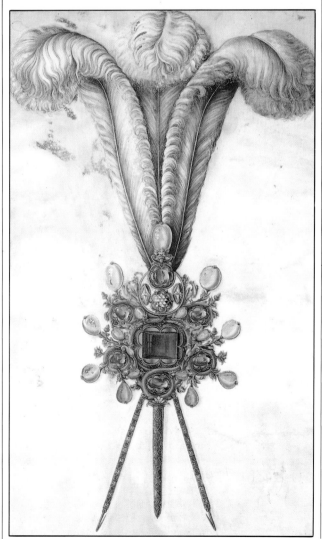

This decorative hat jewel was recorded by Hans Mielich in the pictorial inventory of the collection of Duke Albrecht V of Bavaria and his wife, Duchess Anna. The gemstones and pearls are mounted in a design of oak branches with acorns, enlivened by small figures – pairs of birds, lizards, and dragons – darting between the settings. The raised six-sided collets are engraved and enameled, an innovation of the 1540s.

INTRODUCTION

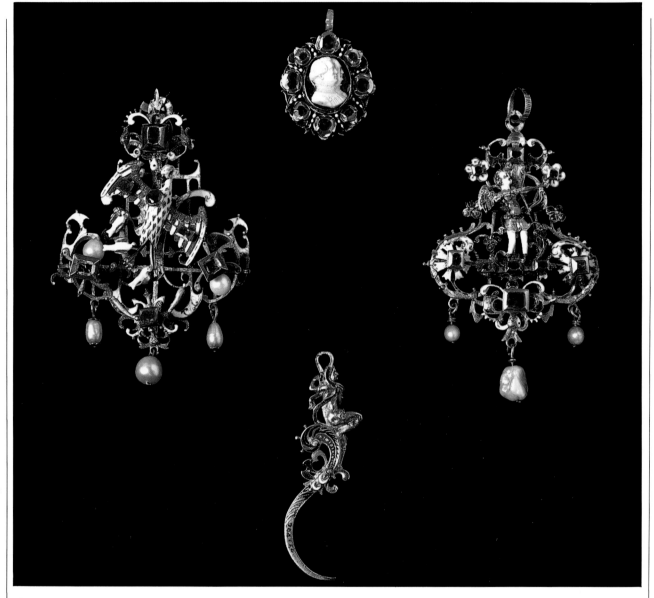

succeeded the elementary point – and table – cut early in the 17th century, and then in the 1660s the brilliant cut became available, releasing more light from the diamond than ever before. To prevent yellow reflections silver settings were substituted for gold, which was then used for colored stones only. Often combined with diamonds, these colored stones were both precious – emeralds, sapphires, and rubies – and semiprecious – amethysts, chrysoberyls, peridots, turquoises, topazes, coral, jet, and opals. Pearls, if white, round and flawless, were more prized than any of these, and were threaded in the hair, hung from the ears, worn next to the skin around the neck and wrists, and set in jewels.

Substitutes for pearls and colored stones could be obtained in Paris and Venice, while colorless crystals which could be faceted were a cheap alternative to diamonds. Not only were figurative elements banished from settings but the role of enamel was much reduced except in watch cases and lockets. Thanks to a technique invented by the Toutin family of Blois, flat surfaces could be enameled with still-life, topographical, and genre scenes and reproductions of the Baroque canvases of Simon Vouet and Charles Lebrun – continuing the 16th-century association between the fine arts and personal ornaments.

Pattern books reflect the contemporary passion for botany and plant life. Balthasar Lemersier's *Bouquets d'Orfèvrerie* (1626) contains variations on the theme of pea-pod plants – called *cosse de pois* – with sprays of leaves shooting upward and curved around petal-shaped settings for gemstones. A more naturalistic style was developed by Johann Paul Hauer in 1650, and then, in tune with the classicism of Versailles, acanthus leaves became a dominant theme.

The Hair Jewels of the Mid–17th Century

In the middle of the 17th century only a few jewels were worn with the hair fashions of the day: the face was framed with ringlets and a string of pearls might be entwined in the chignon and bodkins placed at the sides. These were ornamented with jeweled insects such as butterflies, dragonflies, snails, and caterpillars perched on long stems, or with shepherds' crooks and flowers studded with rose-cut diamonds and cabochon gemstones. In contrast, by the 1690s, large floral sprays with stems bent under the weight of diamonds and pearls emphasized the tall, padded coiffures which were worn with feathers dyed to match the ribbons tied in bows on the dress. The high pleated, stiffened lace "Fontanges" head-dresses, which originated at Versailles, also sparkled with clusters of faceted stones scattered on the front and sides of the head. Men's hats were encircled by bands of gemstones or gold chains and strings of pearls. The aigrette remained in fashion until it was superseded by the button and loop holding up the brim around 1700.

Notwithstanding the immense popularity of pear pearls at this time, some earrings were made of gemstones and goldsmith's work. Amethysts carved into bunches of grapes which probably date from the middle of the century were found in the Cheapside Hoard (the stock of a jeweler discovered on a site in Cheapside in London in 1912), and there must have been other such imaginative designs. Most characteristic of the period is the girandole, consisting of a top cluster with three pendants branching out like the arms of a candelabra and sometimes linked to the main cluster by a ribbon bowknot.

Large natural pearls, evenly matched like peas in a pod, were most sought after for necklaces, which were tied at the back with ribbon bows. But the diamond, with its new brilliance, had asserted its pre-eminence by the time of the coronation of Queen Anne in London in 1702, when many peeresses wore necklaces of rose-cut stones simply set in heavy silver mounts with one or two rows falling in front like festoons. A role was found for enamel on chains and necklaces: some were composed of plaques painted with landscapes and allegorical figures, of blue, black and white bowknots, and red stars, each centered on a pearl.

Men prided themselves on their insignia, jeweled buttons, and miniatures or badges of honor hanging from gold chains. An innovation with a long future ahead of it was the sleeve button, designed to fasten the cuff at each

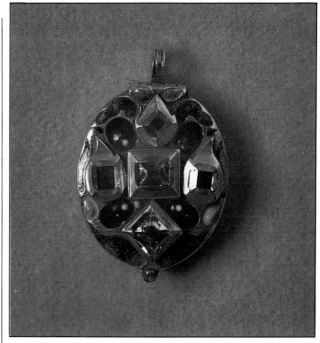

The back of this diamond-studded miniature case, c.1610–20, is enameled with a crowned red heart transfixed by arrows and inscribed in French "Fidel iusq a la mort le pareil de vous a mon confort" ("Faithful unto death your likeness is my comfort").

wrist and replacing the ribbon used until then. These appear in England in the late 1660s.

In the first half of the 17th century women of fashion almost invariably wore a large jewel in the center of the corsage. Hélène Fourment wears a large gold and diamond jewel of *cosse de pois* design with long jeweled stems shooting upward around a central cluster, in a portrait *c.*1630 painted by her husband, Rubens. These, like crosses, might be pinned over a ribbon bowknot, but from the middle of the 17th century the bowknot was interpreted in metal and gemstones, ultimately being combined with acanthus scrolls, following Versailles fashion. Brandenburgs, of oblong form, inspired by the frogging on the jackets of Prussian soldiers and worn as one large jewel or in graduated sets down to the waist, were another Versailles fashion which was taken up internationally. In the interests of a uniformly elegant toilette, brooches, buttons, sleeve clasps, earrings, necklaces, and aigrettes were increasingly being made in sets of matching design and material, evolving into the 18th-century parure.

Two constant themes in 17th-century jewelry were death and politics. The successive constitutional crises in England are evoked by rings, brooches, lockets, and bracelet slides – worn on velvet bands passing through loops at the back – representing Charles I and his children, and then William and Mary. Memorial jewels commemorating private individuals are of similar design: they are ornamented with *memento mori* symbols – skulls and crossbones, hourglasses, and coffins – and often contain locks of hair identified with ciphers worked in gold wire.

INFLUENCES

The architecture of the Italian Renaissance was gradually adopted in northern countries beyond the Alps; in France, for example, François I and Henri II built the palace of Fontainebleau around a series of courts in the classical style, here illustrated in a drawing by Jacques Ducerceau, c. 1570 (**2**). In jewelry, one of the ways in which classicism was expressed was in the revival of the ancient art of engraving hardstones in relief. This sardonyx cameo (**1**) of Omphale wearing the lion-skin of her lover, Hercules, set in a gold jeweled pendant, was given by the Hapsburg emperor Charles V to the Medici pope Clement VII.

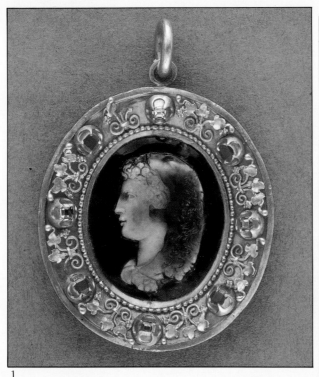

1

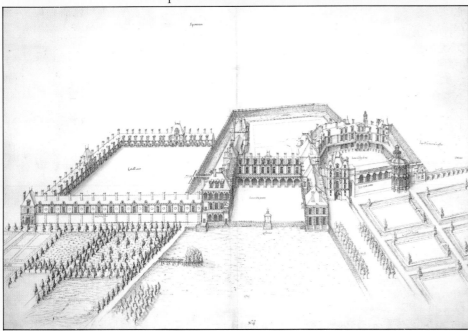

2

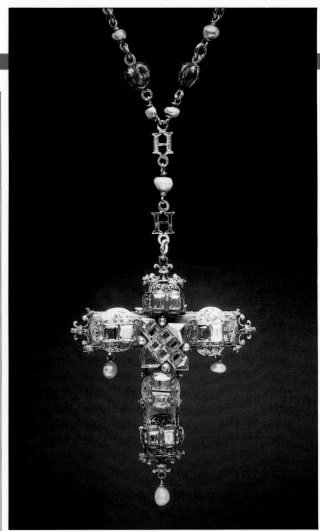

3

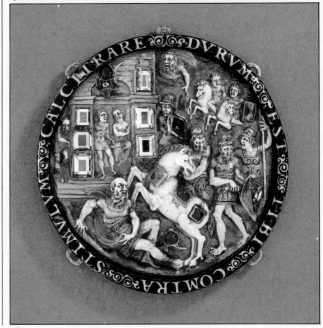

4

54

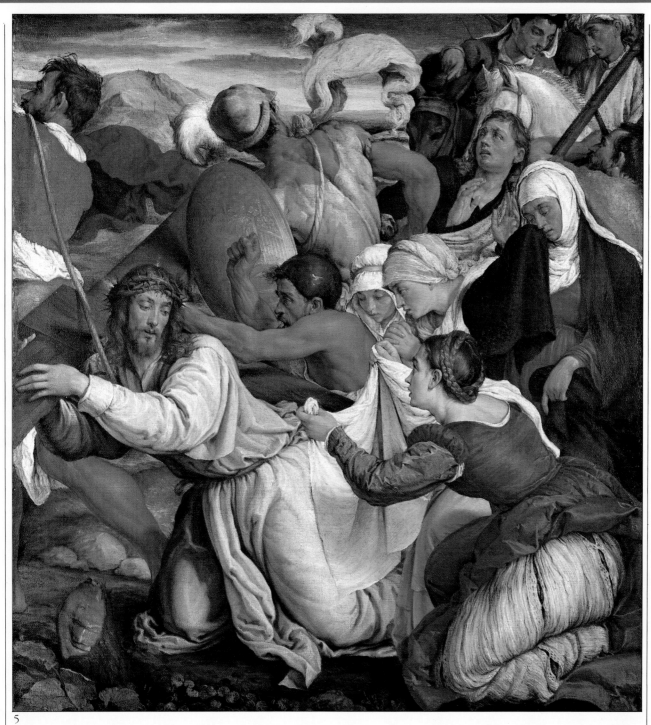

5

The Protestant Reformation did not bring the medieval custom of wearing devotional jewelry to an end. The most powerful of Christian symbols – the cross – was brought up to date: here table-cut diamonds are set in raised quatrefoil collets, whose sides are chased with crescents outlined in enamel (3). Episodes from the Old and New Testaments were wrought in enameled gold, highlighted with gemstones. Don John of Austria is said to have worn this hat badge (4) depicting the Conversion of St Paul, and these miniature jeweled tableaus (5) are the goldsmith's versions of religious paintings such as Jacopo Bassano's Way of Calvary, c. 1540.

PENDANTS AND ACCESSORIES

Illustrating the international court style is a Portuguese crown jewel, a pendent scent bottle in the form of a lion with ruby eyes, jeweled collar, and naturalistically chased mane and coat studded with table- and rose-cut diamonds (*1*). The diamond heart held in the forepaws is inscribed in Italian, "*Qui soggiorna che gire ancor.*" The head unscrews so that the scent can perfume foul air. Scent bottles and pomanders hung from the girdle or on chains around the neck.

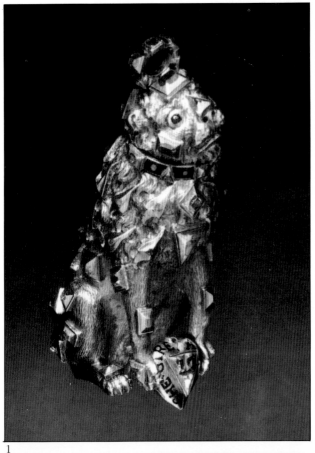

1

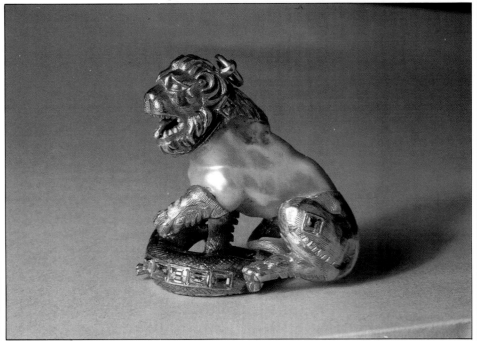

2

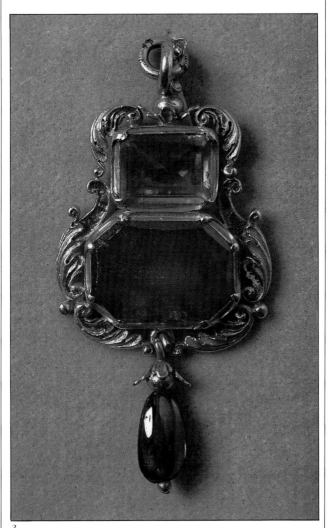

3

The lion with milky-white baroque pearl set in his body contrasts with the gleaming gilt head, forepaws, and hindquarters (*2*). Every gemstone in the Renaissance had a magical property assigned to it. To make sure that the "virtues" of the peridot and hessonite garnet framed in acanthus (*3*) are transmitted directly to the skin, the back of the pendant has been left open.

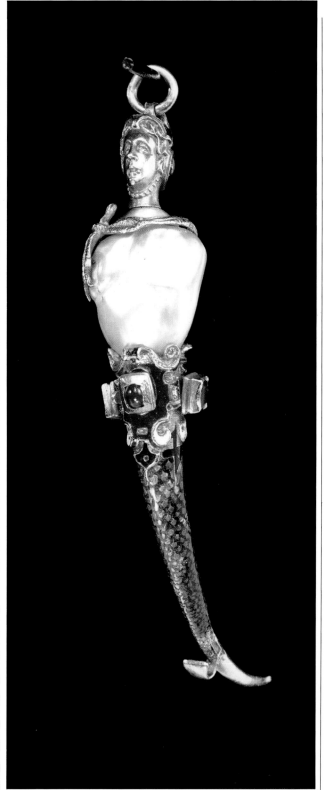

Toothpicks were just as essential to personal comfort as scent and were likewise made into jewels. This mermaid's torso is set with a baroque pearl whose swelling curves simulate feminine contours, and her fish tail is enameled with a green scale-pattern and terminates in the pick (**4**). The sculptural skills of the goldsmith developed so that now several figures could be grouped together in one jewel, often contained in an architectural setting. The Adoration of the Magi is here enacted on a stage framed with ruby obelisks on diamond bases beneath an arch. The diamond star of Bethlehem shines above the Virgin and Child, who are raised on a throne (**5**).

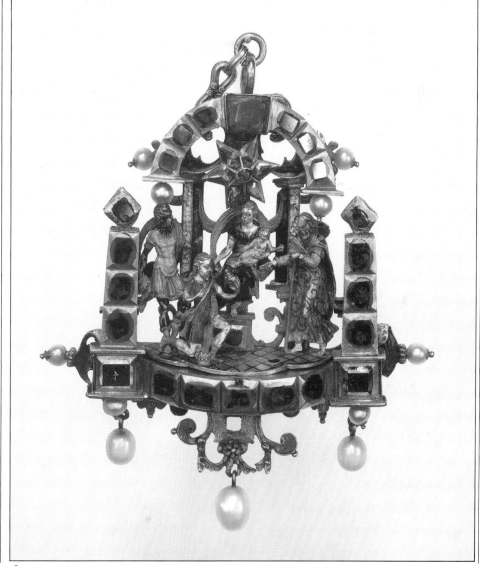

4

5

COLLARS

HANS HOLBEIN

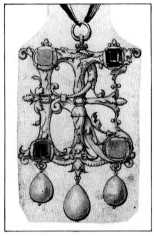 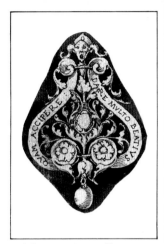

Monogram and lyre pendants of classical character designed by Hans Holbein.

Hans Holbein, in England from 1532 to 1543, designed hat badges, pendants, rings, girdle books, and chains which incorporate classical motifs: masks, cornucopias, acanthus leaves and arabesques. Some of them are figurative, illustrating events from mythology or the Bible, such as the wife of Lot turning into a pillar of salt. Inscriptions give an individual charm to Holbein's designs: a lyre-shaped pendant enclosing flowers is inscribed in Latin "Quam accipere dare multo beatus" ("How much better it is to give than to receive"). Holbein classicized the medieval cipher jewel by entwining it with acanthus leaves: the pendant, in the form of RE, set with colored stones and hung with pearls, may refer to Henry VIII – Enricus Rex. Most of these designs are now in the British Museum and, along with contemporary portraits, are all that we have to tell us of early Tudor court jewelry.

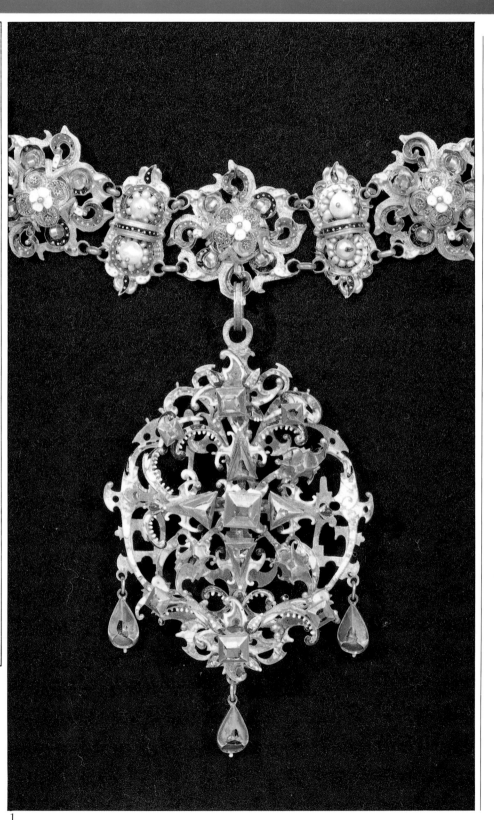

1

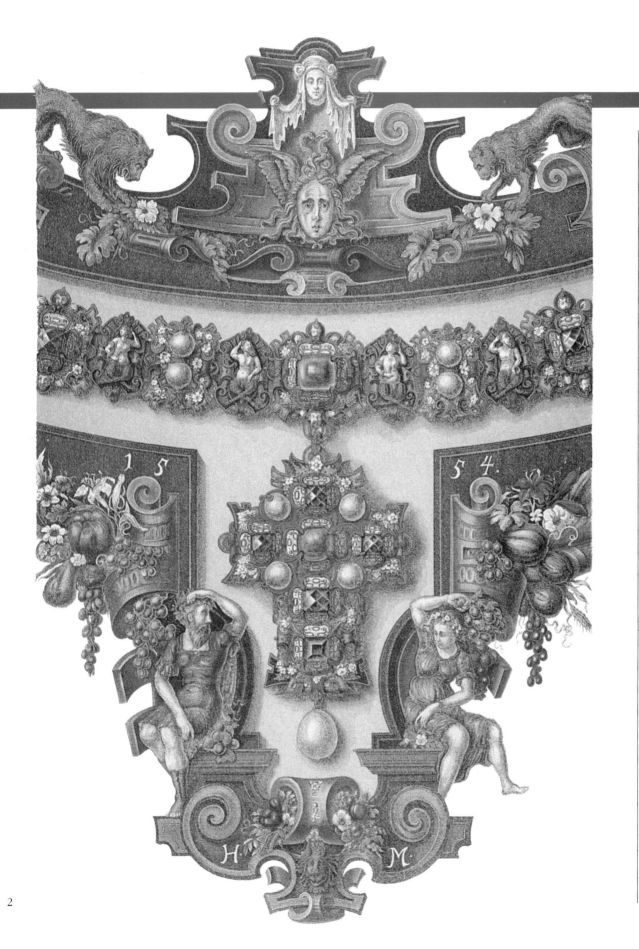

Hans Mielich, court painter to Duke Albrecht V of Bavaria, recorded the jewels of the duke and duchess in a pictorial inventory. One of the grandest of all the magnificent pieces illustrated was this collar (**2**) of wrought gold, enameled in bright colors and set with gemstones alternating with pairs of pearls in floral frames, and with figures of satyrs and nymphs seated in cartouches. Each link is a jewel in its own right. A cross of similar style hangs from the collar with the date 1554. Fifty years later the figurative elements have gone, the enameling is much more sober, and diamonds and pearls play the dominant role in this caracanet and the openwork pendant hanging from it (**1**) from the imperial castle of Ambras. Made by a Hapsburg court jeweler, they illustrate the transition from the figurative style of the Renaissance to the 17th-century emphasis on gemstones.

SENTIMENT IN JEWELRY

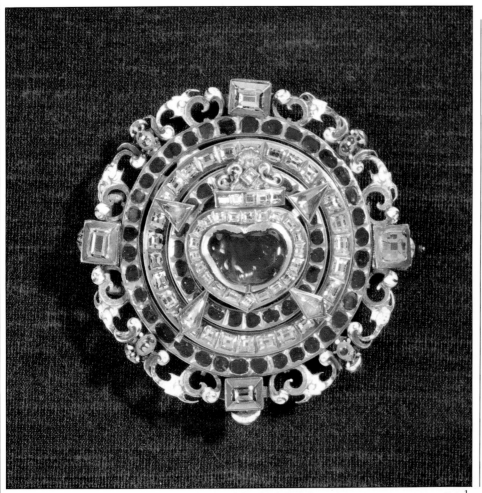

In 17th-century jewelry the heart is used as a religious emblem as well as a sign of personal sentiment. The enameled gold locket (**1**) set with table-cut rubies and diamonds is centered on a ruby heart transfixed by Cupid's arrows and crowned with diamonds – the reward of fidelity. The back (**2**), which is enameled with flowers and leaves, contains the miniature of a man.

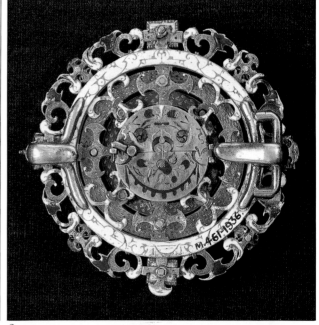

1   2

Representative of the Prague court style, this is said to have belonged to Rakóczy, Prince of Transylvania. An arrow, alluding to Cupid, whose attribute it is, is set with emeralds and rose-cut diamonds; the point, with table-cut garnets, might be worn in the hair (3).

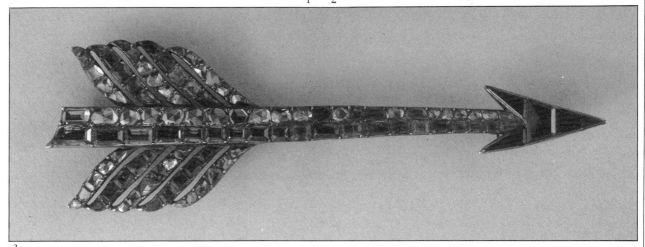

3

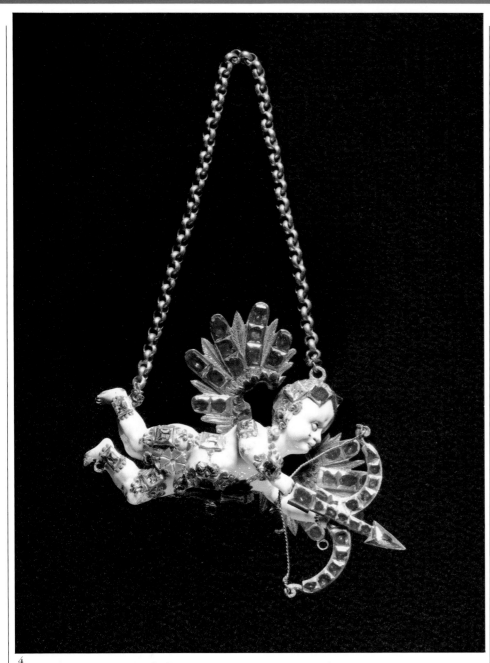

4

Cupid is depicted taking aim with a diamond-tipped arrow and ruby bow in a pendant (**4**) similar to one listed among the jewels of Queen Anna Christina of Denmark in 1597: his body is studded with gemstones, and there is a pearl in his ear.

The heart motif was also adopted for rings and, held by a hand, is applied here (**5**) to the shoulders of a gimmel ring. Gimmel means twin, from the Latin gemellus, and the ring has twin hoops terminating in a double bezel, an allegory of the married state. The hoops are inscribed in Latin with the words from St Matthew's Gospel that affirm the indissolubility of Christian marriage: "Let not man put asunder what God has joined together." The infant and the skeleton in cavities within the bezel refer to man's pilgrimage through life, which he begins as a naked baby and ends when, naked once more, he returns to God (**6**).

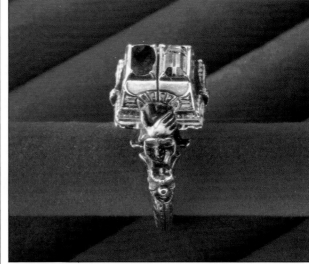

5

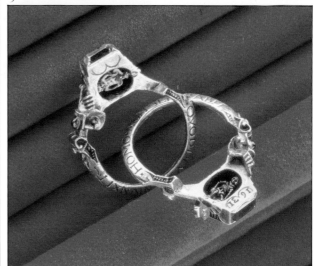

6

BOTANICAL THEMES

Many 17th-century jewels are enameled with patterns of flowers like miniature Dutch still-life paintings. A magnificent watch case (**1**) – probably made for a member of a royal family – with tulips, daisies, and lilies worked in relief in opaque white highlighted with black on a bluish-green ground encloses a movement by the Parisian watchmaker Jehan Cremsdorff. The top cover is set with table-cut diamonds around the circumference converging in six lines on a center stone. Allegorical figures of Charity and Hope ornament the insides of the covers, and there is another on the dial.

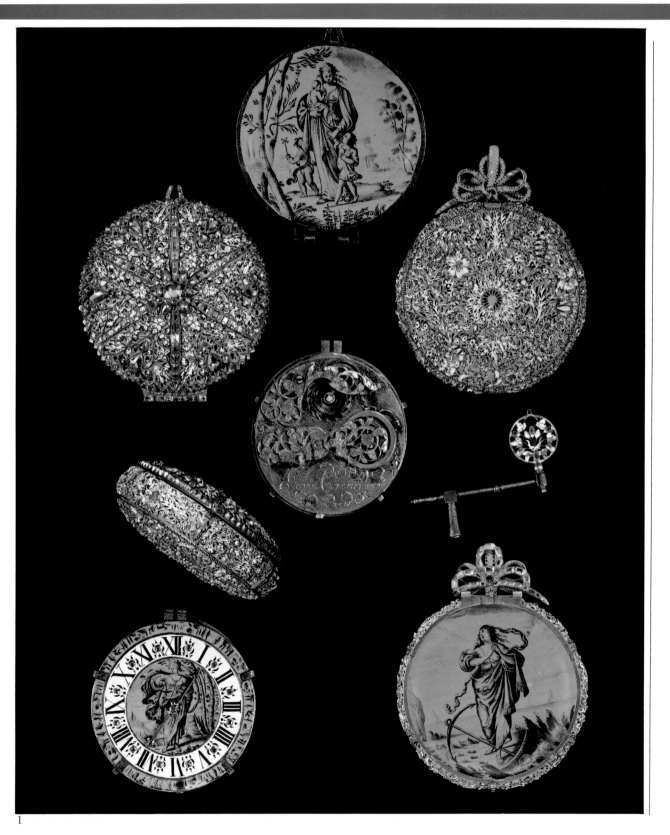

1

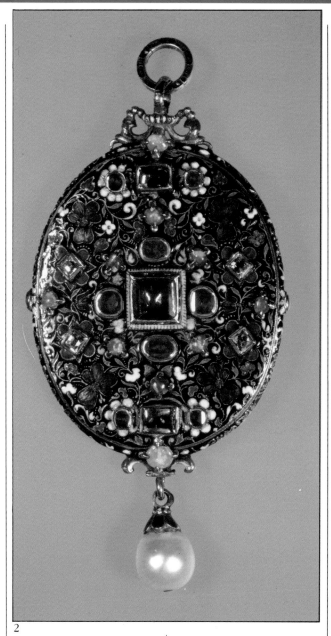

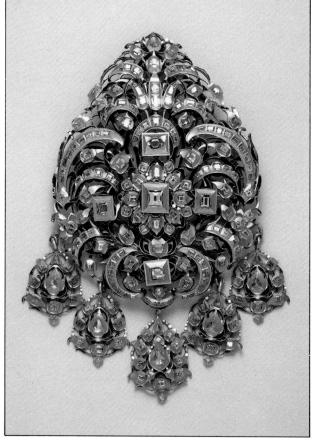

Large numbers of small diamonds are set in a gold cosse de pois (pea-pod)-style breast ornament (3) composed of long-stemmed plants curved around a central cluster, and hung with five pendants. This jewel is close to the designs of Balthasar Lemersier, and in a portrait of c. 1630 Rubens' wife is wearing a similar jewel. Long enameled chains (4) composed of flowers or leaves were among the stock of a mid 17th-century jeweler that was discovered by chance on a site in Cheapside in London in 1912. Of the 35 chains in the board the majority were of floral design.

2

The English court style is illustrated by the enameled gold case (2) containing a miniature of Sir Bevil Grenville who died fighting for Charles I in 1643. The floral pattern stands out brilliantly against the black ground embellished with precious stones.

3

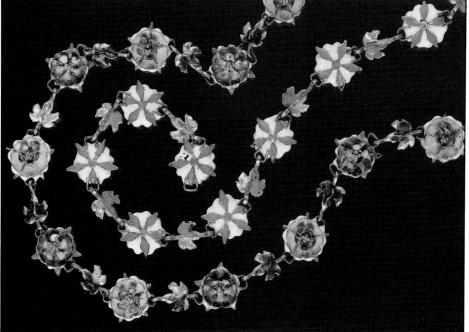

4

DECORATIVE MOTIFS

Inspired by the colored ribbons that trimmed dresses during the 17th century, jewelers created bowknot jewels, most of them for the breast, but also as necklaces with links enameled in opaque colors and centered on a large bowknot studded with diamonds and hung with a sapphire drop (1).

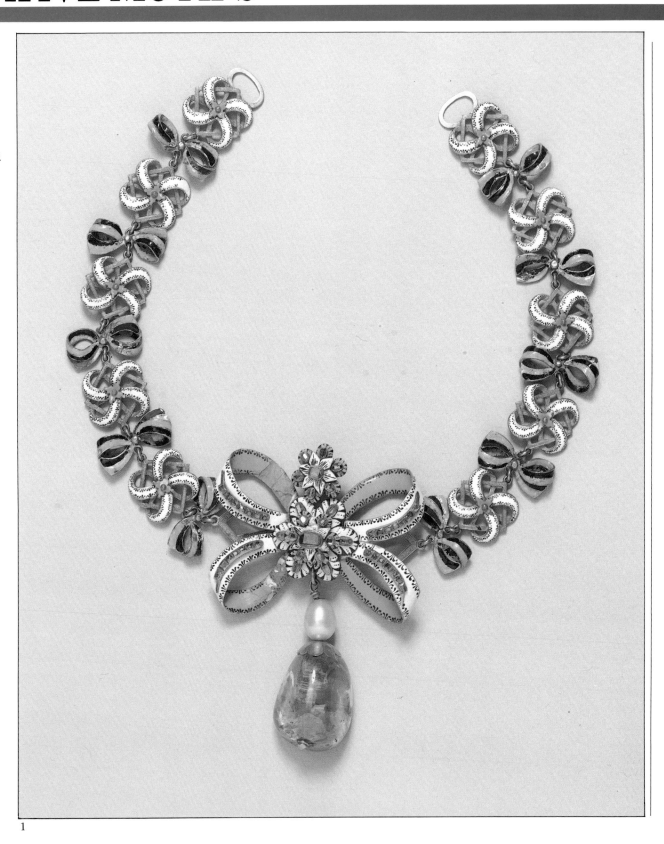

1

MEMENTO MORI

The 17th century was a time of political unrest, long wars, and periodic outbreaks of plague. Religious attitudes and much of literature emphasized the brevity of this life compared with eternity. This was expressed in jewels ornamented with motifs which represented familiar concepts of the passing of time such as the winged hour-glass, coffins, infants blowing bubbles, and skulls and cross bones. In the second half of the century *memento mori* symbols were combined with jewels worn in memory of specific individuals. In England a large category of *memento mori* jewels commemorated King Charles I, executed in 1649, and venerated as a martyr by Royalists.

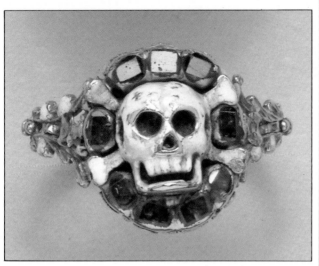

Ring, with skull and crossbones framed in rubies, may have originally been set with diamonds in the eye sockets and nostrils.

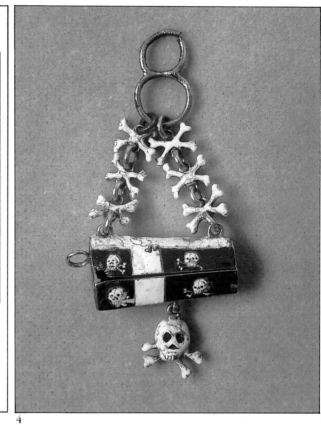

4

In the designs of the itinerant English jeweler Marcus Gunter, acanthus, laden with rose-cut stones and hung with briolettes, is the dominant motif. His aigrette (2) with a long pin to fix in the hair was designed in Amsterdam in 1711; the girandole earrings (3), with triple pendants hanging from the top setting, were made in Siena and are dated 1703.

Crossbones ornament the suspension chains of a coffin pendant (4) enameled and hung with skulls and more crossbones. Inside the coffin a white skeleton is accompanied by the dramatic inscription in German which, translated, means "Here I lie and wait for you I.G.S."

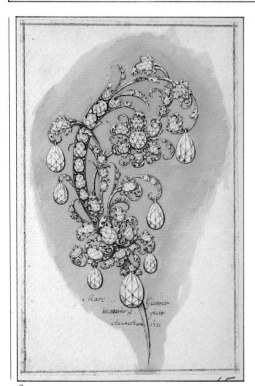

2

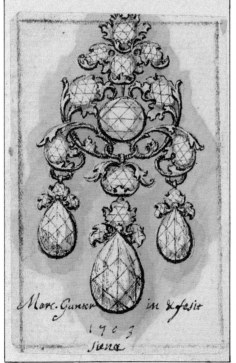

3

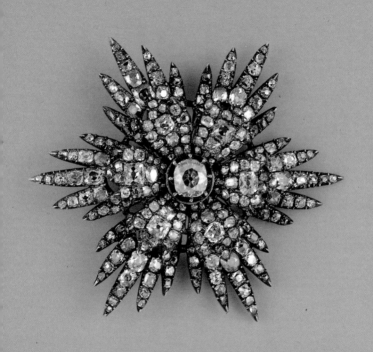

Radiated brooch in stylized flower shape, diamonds set in silver, dated c. 1770

CHAPTER FOUR

ELEGANCE AND ROMANTICISM

1715-1836

The Georgians

·

The Rococo movement

·

The Napoleonic Empire

·

Neoclassicism and revivals

DIANA SCARISBRICK

INTRODUCTION

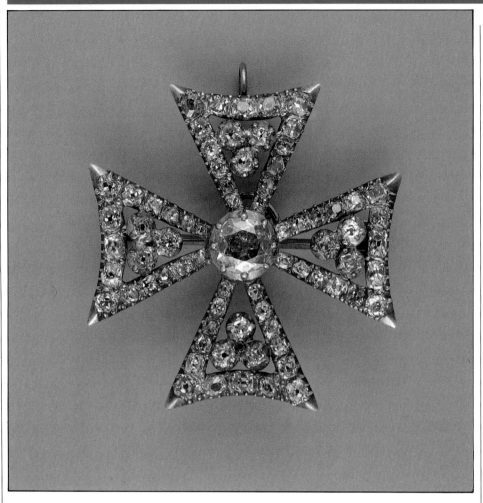

The badge of the Knights of St John of Jerusalem, rulers of the island of Malta from 1530. The Maltese cross was adopted by jewelers in London after the confirmation of British sovereignty by the Treaty of Paris in 1814. Set with diamonds, this cross would have hung from a necklace similarly set, or from a velvet ribbon .

A distinction was made at the beginning of the 18th century between the jewels worn with informal daytime clothes and the grander ornaments – or parures – required with full dress. Since better lighting made it possible for important social occasions to take place at night, "dress" jewels were designed to look their best by candlelight.

The emphasis on stones rather than settings continued to increase, and improved faceting showed off the full beauty of diamonds and colored stones in lighter, more informal and delicate designs in tune with the elegant rococo spirit. The traditional source of gemstones in India was supplemented by imports of diamonds from Brazil, eclipsing pearls, though these were still much worn. Not only sparkle was expected of jewels, but also deep flashes of color, achieved by expert foiling, while some jewelers, notably G.F. Strass of Paris, successfully tinted diamonds. France remained the fount of inspiration for style and craftsmanship, which were upheld abroad by the Huguenots and by Parisian jewelers invited to work at foreign courts: J.F. Fistaine in Copenhagen, Louis Duval in St Petersburg, and Augustin Duflos in Madrid. Engravings by designers such as Mondon and Pouget diffused French fashions further, and since clients everywhere acknowledged their superiority, fine jewelry was international in character.

Seventeenth-century designs were brought up to date: aigrettes and ornamental insects – moths, flies, and butterflies – for the hair, girandole earrings, bowknots for the bodice. Acanthus was discarded, asymmetry was introduced, and ribbonwork became more fluid and intricate, interspersed with flowers. This naturalistic trend continued into the late Georgian period, then after 1761 Neo-classical fret (or key pattern), honeysuckle, and husks appear, contained in compact geometrical forms which, although more severe, still have the elegance of the rococo. Enamel disappears from the backs of settings, which from the 1760s are backed with gold, thus preventing tarnish.

It is in daytime jewelry that enamel finds a continuing role, decorating chatelaines, watch and miniature cases, lockets, and bracelet clasps. From the 1760s a distinctive blue was used to outline settings and cover the plaques for ciphers on bracelets and rings, the rich color contrasting well with the bright gold luster. Memorial and sentimental jewelry was another daytime favorite. Hair, braided or worked into mesh-like patterns, was incorporated into brooches, rings, bracelet clasps, and pendants hung from chains at the neck, identified with ciphers and framed in small pearls or enameled borders sometimes inscribed with loving messages such as "inséparable jusqu'à la mort." From the 1770s the fichu at the neck might be fastened with an oval-shaped brooch with a love motif: flaming torches, twinned hearts, padlocks, Cupid himself.

Naturalistic sprigs of flowers were placed in the hair and also birds, paved with diamonds and pecking at berries or holding out emerald olive branches. Much to Neo-classical taste in the latter half of the 18th century were jeweled stars, crescents, feathers, and, later, tiaras, which were worn over the brow in the manner of a Roman empress. The large hats then fashionable were pinned with brooches, some themselves designed as miniature hats ornamented with trophies of love and of the arts.

Whether she was in "dress" or "undress," earrings were essential to the appearance of the well-dressed woman. Suitable for day wear were clusters made from cheap materials, especially *coq de perle* from periwinkle shells, and paste in colors matching the dress or trimmings, sold *en suite* with a demi-parure brooch or cross. For evening the elaborate girandole, with its triple pendants, now linked to the top by ribbonwork with flowers, remained a favorite, and single-drop earrings grew to two inches (five centimeters) in length, balancing hair worn high and topped with nodding plumes.

Diamonds were reserved for evening necklaces, and the *rivière* of graduated stones was the most prestigious of all designs. Smaller stones were worked into intricate garlands of flowers and ribbons with an esclavage, or long loop, hanging down from the section encircling the neck. Simpler styles were composed of clusters in rows or jeweled bowknots sewn on a velvet choker worn high on the throat. From the 1770s new motifs were derived from curtain and upholstery trimmings: lines of stones hanging in festoons or set in pendent tassels.

Courtly Jewels

Eighteenth-century court dress was embellished with magnificent stomachers filling the space between the neckline and the waist. The scale presented a challenge to jewelers, who created the large bouquets and bowknots simulating floral-patterned ribbons which are

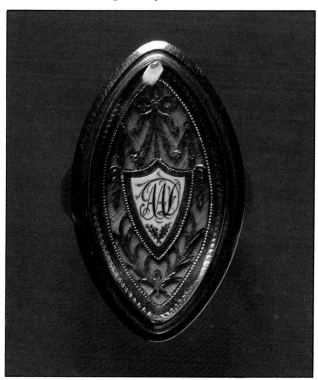

the great triumphs of rococo craftsmanship. Smaller brooches made *en suite* were pinned to the sleeves or scattered over the skirt, their glittering effect enhanced by the rich fabric underneath.

The same high standard of fashionable design and quality was applied to jewels of less expensive materials: bright red carnelian, moss-agate, and garnets, which were foiled to glow like warm rose-red rubies. Substitutes widely used included pinchbeck, a gilt metal invented by a Fleet Street watchmaker, and paste. White and colored paste was almost universally used for buttons, and for buckles on shoes, garters and belts. In Switzerland, where diamonds were forbidden by the sumptuary laws, marcasite was cut into small stones, faceted and polished to shine attractively by candlelight. From the 1760s marcasite was combined with cut steel, a specialty of Matthew Boulton of Birmingham, who exported it all over Europe in chatelaines, pendants, bracelets, brooches, belt clasps, earrings, dress combs, and buttons. Cut steel also combined well with Staffordshire enamels and with the ceramic plaques made by Josiah Wedgwood representing characters and events from antiquity as well as from contemporary literature and history – the white figures standing out in relief against the tinted ground like cameos. Another cheap, mass-produced material used extensively for rings and bracelets was the colored-glass paste made by the Scot James Tassie reproducing ancient and modern engraved gems.

The 18th-century man of fashion also delighted in jewelry. While the privileged few had their magnificent insignia of the Orders of Chivalry for court dress, all gentlemen might expect to carry a sword with jeweled hilt and wear good rings, a fine watch with wrought-gold seal, and a locket or miniature hanging from a chain around the neck. A jeweled pin held the cravat in place, sleeve links fastened the cuffs, and there were paste or cut-steel buckles on shoes, garters, and belt. Buttons – in sets – were essential for the well-trimmed suit, and these – enameled or set with gems or paste – might also indicate cultural and sporting interests. As dress became plainer after the 1770s, so did buttons become excessively large.

The Emergence of Neo-classicism

A simplification of dress, with correspondingly less emphasis on jewelry, marked the years of political change following the French Revolution of 1789, whose effects were felt throughout Europe. However, the emergence of Napoleon as Emperor of France in 1804 brought about a revival in the art of jewelry, as he determined to outshine his Bourbon predecessors by pomp and display. The rich Neo-classical Empire style devised for this purpose by the painter David was applied to the creation of fabulous parures worn by the women of the imperial family on numerous state occasions. Their tiaras, earrings, necklaces, bracelets, and brooches of Greek fret, honeysuckle, palmettes, and wreaths of vine and laurel, studded with diamonds, emeralds, rubies, and engraved gems from the former royal collection, set the standard for the rest of Europe. Although the classical motifs were rejected by the Bourbons after their return to power in 1815, the rich style was not, and the Napoleonic parures were transformed into the equally grandiose scrolled and botanical designs of the Restoration. These were also emulated abroad, particularly in England, where

J. J. Rousseau's novel, La Nouvelle Héloïse *(1761), exalting sentiment and virtue in contrast to the artificiality of fashionable life, promoted the wearing of sentimental jewelry, particularly by day. This shuttle-shaped ring contains a lock of hair identified by a cipher.*

INTRODUCTION

The French painter Jacques Louis David devised an artistic style for Napoleon's Empire which was derived from antiquity. This diadem, which is composed of enameled bay leaves with pearl berries linked by diamond stars, is centered on a paste cameo of a Bacchante and is an inexpensive version of Napoleonic classicizing jewelry.

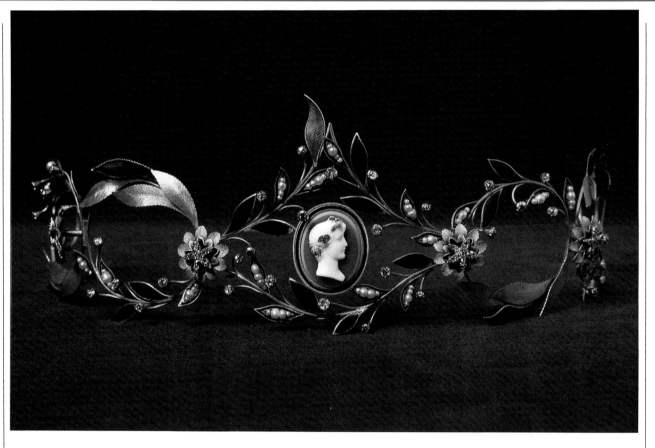

the luxury-loving aristocracy followed the lead of the Prince Regent –later George IV – who had a passion for the superb and magnificent and bought more jewels than any English monarch since Henry VIII.

So great was the desire for huge stones that the supply of precious gemstones had to be supplemented by semi-precious ones. A smart woman might own several parures: violet amethysts, olive-green peridots, golden and pink topazes, apple-green chrysoprases, light blue aquamarines, greenish-yellow chrysoberyls, and brilliant blue turquoises, set in showy mounts of filigree or stamped gold linked by chains. The combination of brightly colored stones in gold settings was called *à l'antique*.

While these grand Empire and Restoration styles were reserved for formal occasions, a wide range of other jewels expressing personal sentiment, patriotism, and nostalgia for the past were worn informally with the picturesque clothes that went with Romanticism, now in full swing. Inspired by popular Romantic novels like those of Sir Walter Scott, women of fashion wore jewels evoking the vanished world of the Middle Ages and Renaissance – representing knights in armor or romantic figures such as Raphael and his mistress. Dining with the Archduchess Marie-Louise, Napoleon's widow, on a visit to Verona in

1822, the poet Châteaubriand was astonished to see on her wrists not rows of diamonds and rubies but bracelets made from marble chipped off the tomb of Shakespeare's heroine Juliet, who was supposedly buried in the city.

In 1839 the *World of Fashion* magazine observed "the forms of our bijoux are now entirely borrowed from the Middle Ages." This was particularly true of devotional jewelry worn as a consequence of the religious revival which accompanied Romanticism, especially in Europe. Belt buckles – large so as to emphasize the fashionable small waist – might represent pilgrims kneeling at a Romanesque shrine; crosses of Greek, Latin, Maltese, and Jerusalem design were ornamented with cusping and tracery; rosaries and rosary rings were proudly displayed for the first time since the Renaissance.

This is also the golden age of sentimental jewelry, with locks of hair, and miniatures – sometimes of the loved one's eye alone – framed in jeweled lockets worn at the neck, wrist, and fingers. The snake, tail in mouth, making a full circle and signifying eternity, is the most representative motif of the period, and is wrought into necklaces, bracelets, pendants, and rings. Hearts and padlocks are ornamented with flowers – the forget-me-not and the pansy – carrying a specific message, while other messages might be spelt out from the initials of the stones used, REGARD (Ruby, Emerald, Garnet, Amethyst, Diamond), AMITIE, SOUVENIR and Christian names being some of the most usual.

Hair and Neck Jewels

The formality of social life required jewels for the hair, and every great lady now wore a tiara with ostrich plumes, *en suite* with a jeweled comb which kept the tall coiffure in place. Smaller bouquets of flowers, ears of wheat, butterflies, and moths were also worn on the side of the head, mounted with trembler springs to heighten the illusion of realism. In 1830 the *ferronière* appeared, inspired by a portrait in the Louvre attributed to Leonardo da Vinci of a lady beloved by Francois I who was also a blacksmith's wife, hence her name, La Belle Ferronière. Simple or splendid according to the occasion, the *ferronière* is always centered on an ornament over the brow, perhaps a cameo, or a drop, or a large cabochon stone. Equally picturesque were the toques and turbans –evoking the Crusades – which were pinned with crescent and feather brooches.

Piled-up hair was balanced by long earrings, made *en suite* with the crosses or brooches that were pinned to the center of the low neckline. The girandole style was still a favorite, but more characteristic of the period were single elongated pendants. In England these might be framed with wreaths of laurel alluding to the victories of the navy and army over Napoleon.

Much of the elegance of 18th-century necklace design was retained, notwithstanding the desire for rich display. Clusters - single stones framed by smaller ones - were linked by groups of diamonds and might be fringed with pendants hanging below. Chains or *sautoirs,* worn across the bosom, were hooked in at the waist and terminated in brightly colored Geneva watches, large crosses, vinaigrettes or lorgnettes. The links might be composed of enameled plaques with seed pearls but more usually were wrought from gold or pinchbeck, each fastened with a clasp shaped like a woman's hand, beringed and braceleted.

Bracelets - broad bands with important clasps - had always been included in parures, but were now worn in rows up the arm from wrist to elbow, in many different designs. They might be in the Gothic style, with traceried arches, or represent a snake with its coils wound several times around the wrist and a heart-shaped locket in its mouth. For clasps the Tudor rose was a favorite in England, with its historical and patriotic associations, and everywhere the motif of two hands clasped - revived from the Renaissance - was adopted for engagement presents.

In spite of the very marked concentration on jewelry for women in this period, the dandy with his gold chains and jeweled studs, pins, rings, and lockets kept the tradition of masculine ornaments very much alive.

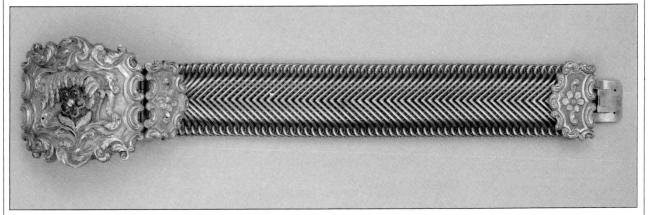

The billowing sleeves of a Romantic period dress were covered from wrist to elbow with wide bracelets. The prominent clasps might be set with an important stone or, as here, wrought in gold, deeply chased with burnished scrolls and leaves on a matte ground, and hinged, opening to a miniature inside.

INFLUENCES

Madame de Pompadour was known for her exquisite taste and, as mistress of Louis XV, could command the greatest artistic talents of France. In a portrait (*3*) by François Boucher, her favorite painter, she epitomizes 18th-century elegance. She was also the patroness of the gem engraver Jacques Guay and commissioned cameos and intaglios from him for bracelet clasps. The subjects usually refer to contemporary French history.

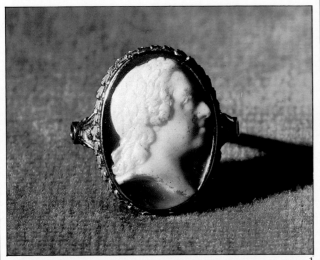

1

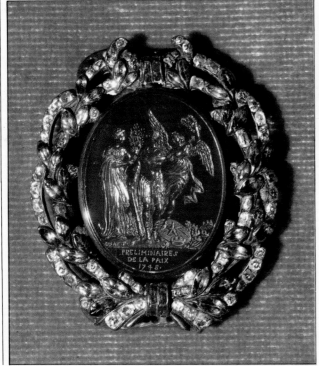

2

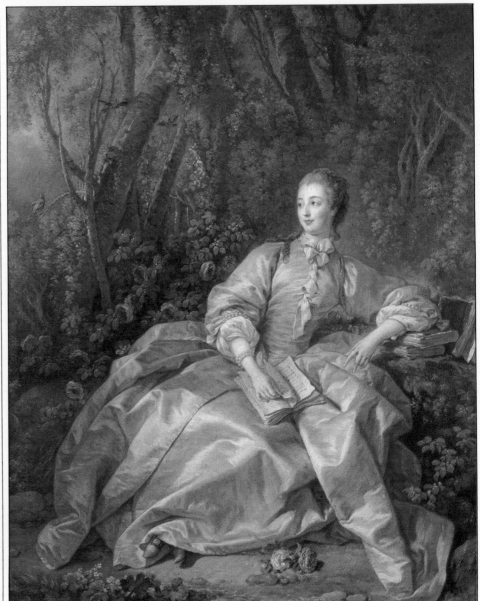

3

This cornelian intaglio (*2*) of Louis XV as Hercules between Victory and Peace, is inscribed "Préliminaires de la paix 1748." Framed in diamond olive branches, it fastened Madame de Pompadour's pearl bracelet. She learned to cut cameos herself, and the portrait of Louis XV is her own work which she wore in a ring (*1*).

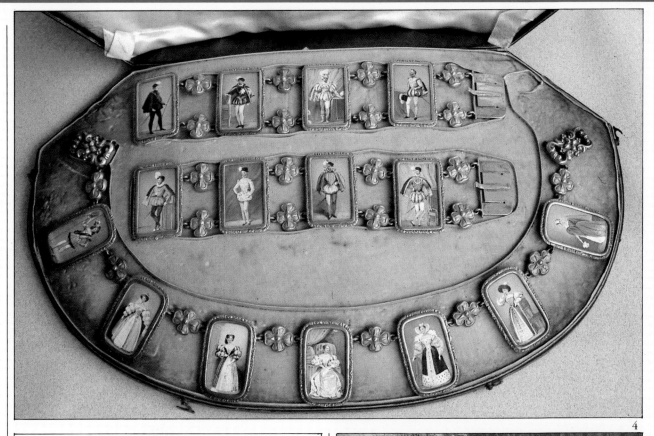

4

Nostalgia for the Middle Ages and the Renaissance was an aspect of Romanticism which found expression in costume balls, where guests impersonated historical characters. One of the most famous of such events was the Quadrille Mary Stuart held at the Tuileries by the Duchesse de Berri in 1829, when a visit of Mary of Guise from Scotland to the court of François II and her daughter Mary Stuart in 1559 was re-enacted. An album of watercolors by Eugène Lami recorded the costumes (6), and the duchess was given a necklace and pair of bracelets enameled with miniatures of some of the most successful (4). In London the Marchioness of Londonderry opened Holdernesse House with a costume ball, where, dressed as Queen Elizabeth and covered with jewels, she greeted her guests seated on a throne (5).

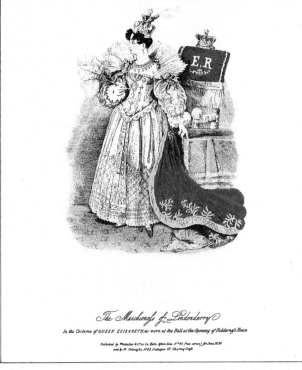

The Marchioness of Londonderry

In the Costume of QUEEN ELIZABETH, as worn at the Ball at the Opening of Holderness House

Published by Whittaker & Co., La Belle Assemblée, No. 56 (new series) for June, 1830 and by M. Colnaghi, No. 23, Cockspur St. Charing Cross

5

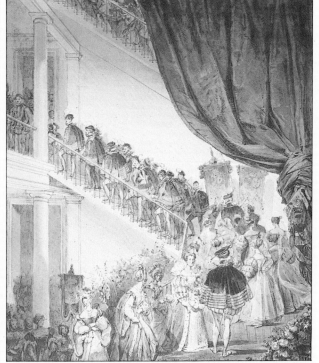

6

RINGS

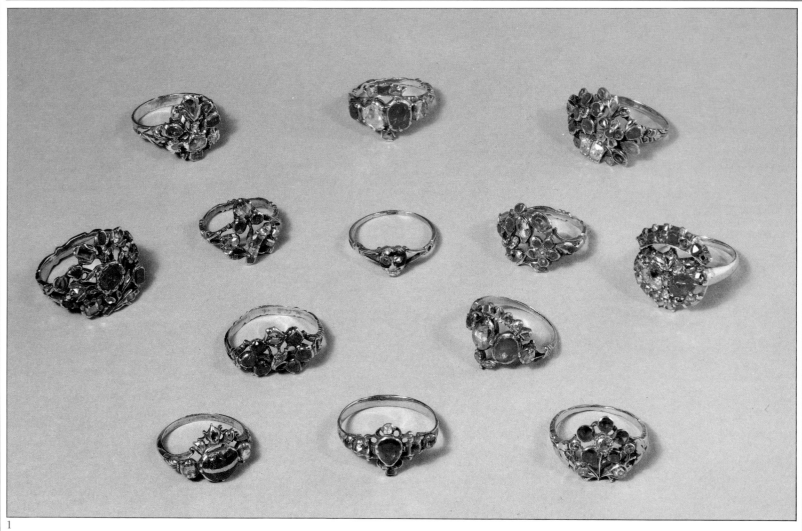

1

Rings provided the final touch of elegance to the toilette. This group includes openwork sprays of flowers, tied with ribbons or placed in a vase, set with small rose-cut diamonds or colored stones, known as "giardinetti" or "gardens." Love rings are designed around the heart motif: single, twinned, bound together by a golden band, and crowned with diamonds. The enameled carnival mask center recalls one of the favorite amusements of 18th-century society, the masquerade or masked ball (1). In contrast to these light-hearted trifles Neo-classical rings are more solid and serious. Here, the golden figure of Diana on a lapis-blue ground derives from a famous intaglio at Naples signed by the Roman court engraver Dioscourides, and the polished sardonyx is a perfect specimen, resembling an eye (2).

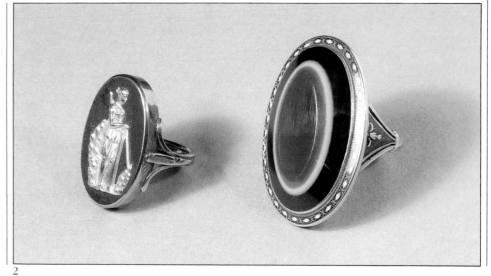

2

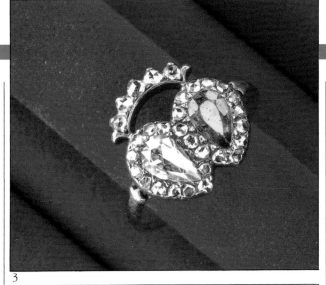

3

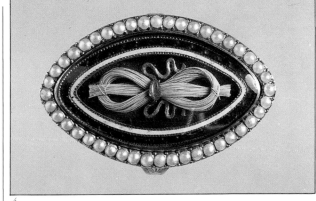

4

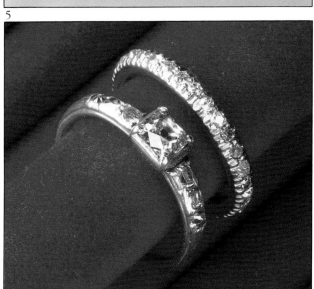

5

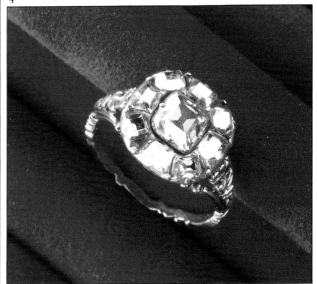

6

7

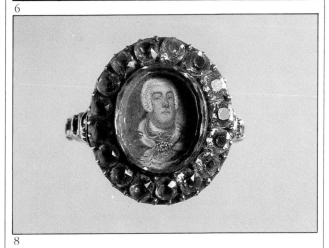

8

Another hardstone much admired was moss-agate, with inclusions simulating the branches of trees or even landscapes, which was set in rings and framed in diamonds (**5**). Love rings were set not only with ruby hearts (**1**) but also with emeralds contrasting with diamonds and bound together and crowned (**3**). The wedding ring was usually a gold band with a love poem or nosegay inside, which might be protected by a keeper, such as the diamond hoop worn by Queen Charlotte, wife of George III, of which this (**7**) is a copy. Diamonds might be set in rows (**7**) or in cluster bezels (**6**) supported by gold hoops which divided at the shoulders and sometimes enclosed a leaf or flower. Miniatures were now small enough to wear in rings: that of Augustus the Strong, King of Poland and Elector of Saxony, is richly framed in diamonds (**8**). Neo-Classical sentiment, which developed under the influence of Jean Jacques Rousseau, was expressed in large rings containing the hair of a loved one, living or dead, framed in deep blue and white borders and rimmed with pearls (**4**).

ROCOCO FLOWERS

Flowers are the principal theme in rococo jewelry, as they are in the other decorative arts of the period. French designers, such as J. H. Pouget, in Traité des Pierres Précieuses (1762), published many designs for floral jewels. A choker (**1**) consists of a garland of colored pastes – even the richest women did not spurn paste.

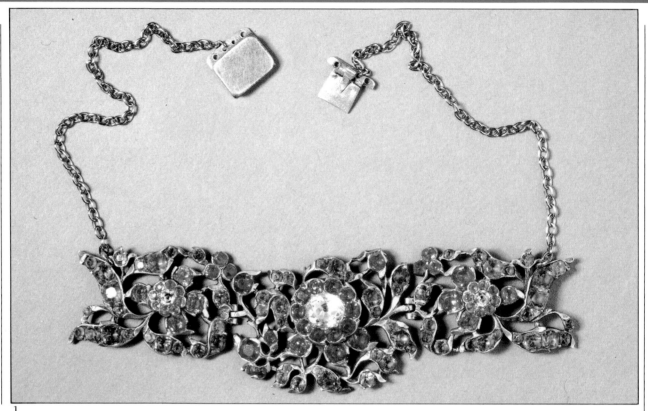

1

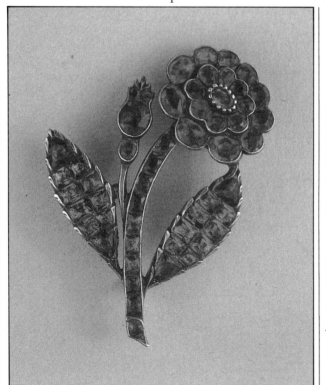

2

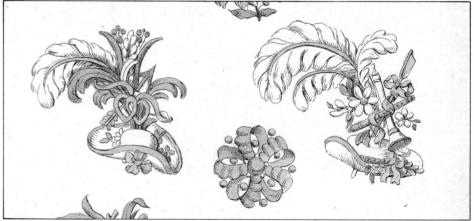

3

Expert foiling produced colors such as the deep red and green in the single flower brooch (**2**). Some delightful creations are hat brooches pinned with sprays of flowers combined with feathers and trophies of love and music (**3**).

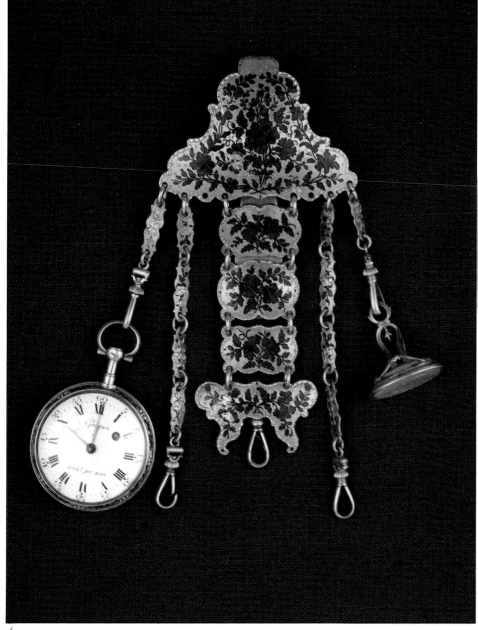

4

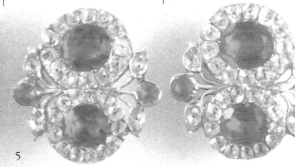

Sprays of flowers and leaves might soften the favorite double cluster style of earring (5) which lit up the face from the sides.

5

Sometimes enamel was combined with gemstones, as in a large, realistically modeled bouquet (6) donated to the Sanctuary of the Virgin of the Pillar at Saragossa (by Dona Juana Rabasa). The deep blue bouquets and festoons

enameled on the bookplate and suspension chains of an English chatelaine of c. 1760 make a striking contrast with the bright gold ground (4).

6

RUBIES AND GARNETS

Color, which was such an important element in 18th-century jewelry, was provided by precious stones, enamel, and paste. The warm red of rubies is enhanced by the white light of diamonds in a pair of bracelets (**1**) composed of two rows of clusters between lines of diamonds.

An equally effective contrast is provided less expensively by garnets and lemon-yellow chrysolites or topazes which enliven an aigrette (**3**) worn to the side of tall padded hair and pinned to nodding ostrich plumes.

Equally successful is the combination of rubies, topazes, emeralds, and diamonds in a pair of girandole earrings (**2**), the triple drops linked by leafy sprays of flowers. Under the patronage of the empresses of Russia, the jewelers of St Petersburg created such rich interpretations of the rococo style as the ruby and diamond spray (**4**) made in c. 1750–1770, which is a tour de force of setting, for the stones have been massed together in a mosaic of color and light with almost no metal showing.

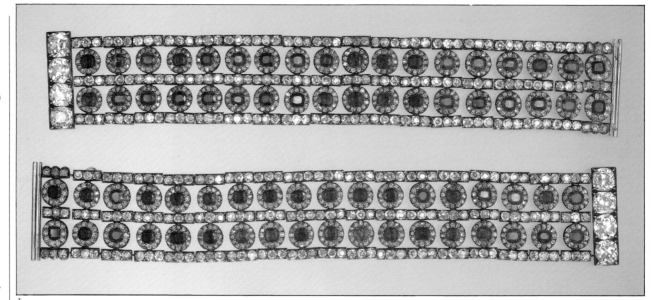

1

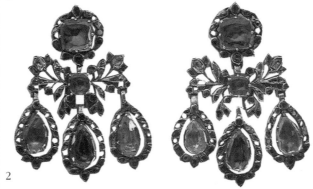

2

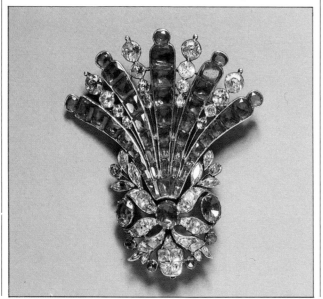

3

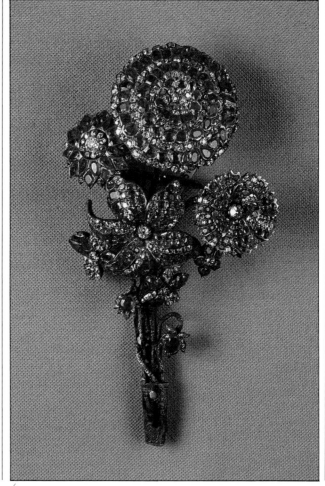

4

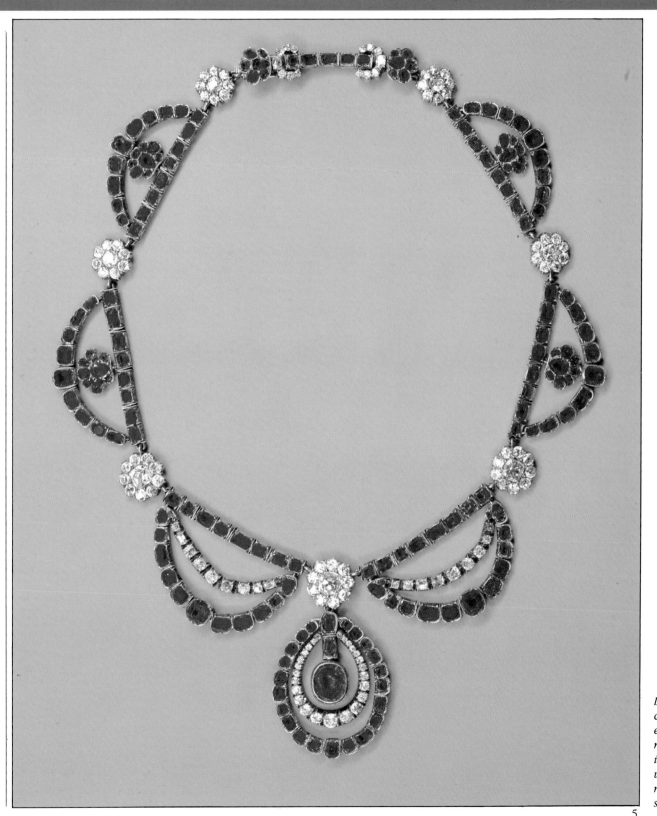

Low necklines were de rigueur *for court dress and left space for elegant compositions such as this ruby and diamond necklace (**5**) intersected by clusters and hung with festoons culminating in a ruby pendant. The diamonds are set in silver, the rubies in gold.*

5

ROMANTICISM

Glass mosaic and gold parure of necklace, comb, and earrings (belt clasp missing) c. 1810. The medallions represent Pompeian bird and butterfly motifs and a spaniel in a landscape, and were a Roman specialty, being made by craftsmen trained in the Vatican work-shops making murals and floors in the ancient tradition. Like cameos engraved in hardstone or shell, glass mosaic jewelry was acquired by visitors as a souvenir of travel (**1**).

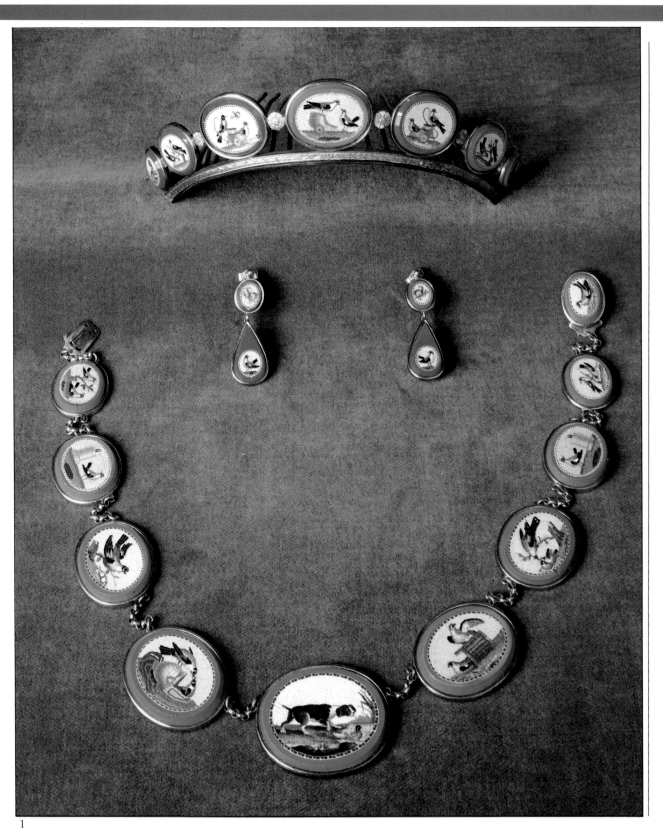

1

Regional Specialities

Coral carved into beads or cameos could be bought in Naples and Genoa; and in Florence, ornaments inlaid with hardstones in decorative patterns. North of the Alps the Swiss excelled at enameling. Watchcases and chains sold well, but it was the bracelets composed of plaques showing young women dressed in the costumes of the respective cantons which most appealed to British travelers, who compared these with the drab agricultural and urban workers' dress at home. Ivory carving of sporting

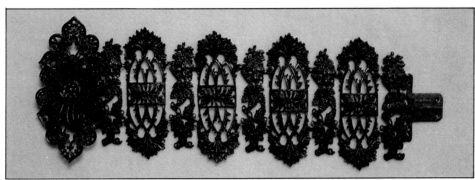

Berlin Iron Gothic Revival bracelet c. 1830.

subjects came from the Black Forest: these were made up into earrings, bracelets, and brooches. From Berlin came severe black ornaments cast in the foundries in classical designs with honeysuckle, fret, and molded replicas of cameos. After 1820 Gothic ornament – ogival arches, rose windows, and trefoils – predominate.

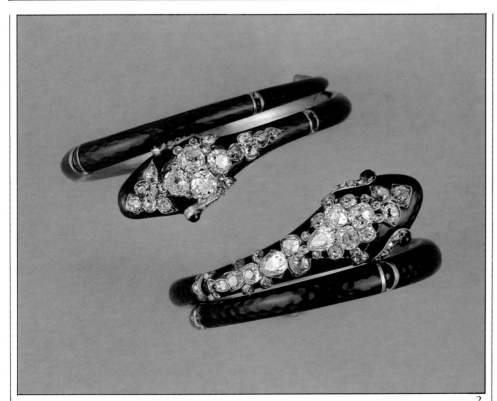

2

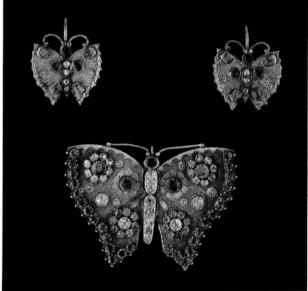

3

The snake, emblem of eternity and symbol of wisdom, was worn by both men and women in jewels during the Romantic period and after. The coils looked good around the arm in bracelets, enameled blue, with diamond heads and ruby eyes (2).

Eighteenth-century naturalism never went out of fashion, but was transformed into richer, more colorful compositions such as this demi-parure (3) of brooch and earrings, the gemstones being set in bright yellow gold "antique style."

ROMANTICISM

Crowned emperor in 1806, Napoleon sought to impose his authority by a great show of pomp and luxury. Such was his success that after the Restoration of 1815 the Bourbon monarchy – who also wished to impress and command respect – adopted the same grandiose style of jewelry, with large stones set in substantial mounts, unambiguously declaring wealth and status. This is the background to the necklace of a graduated double row of sapphires set round with diamonds, worn with earrings en suite (*1*). For daytime wear long chains were hung across the shoulders and hooked at the waist with a watch or lorgnette. They were usually made of pinchbeck with links of different designs stamped with stars. This chain (*2*) is fastened by a pair of hands, beringed and emerging from rose-patterned cuffs.

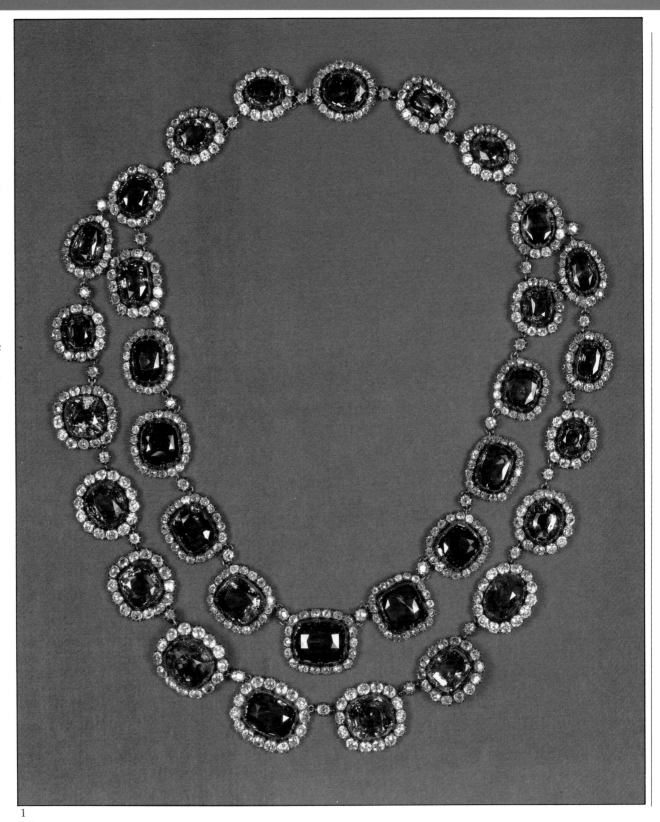

1

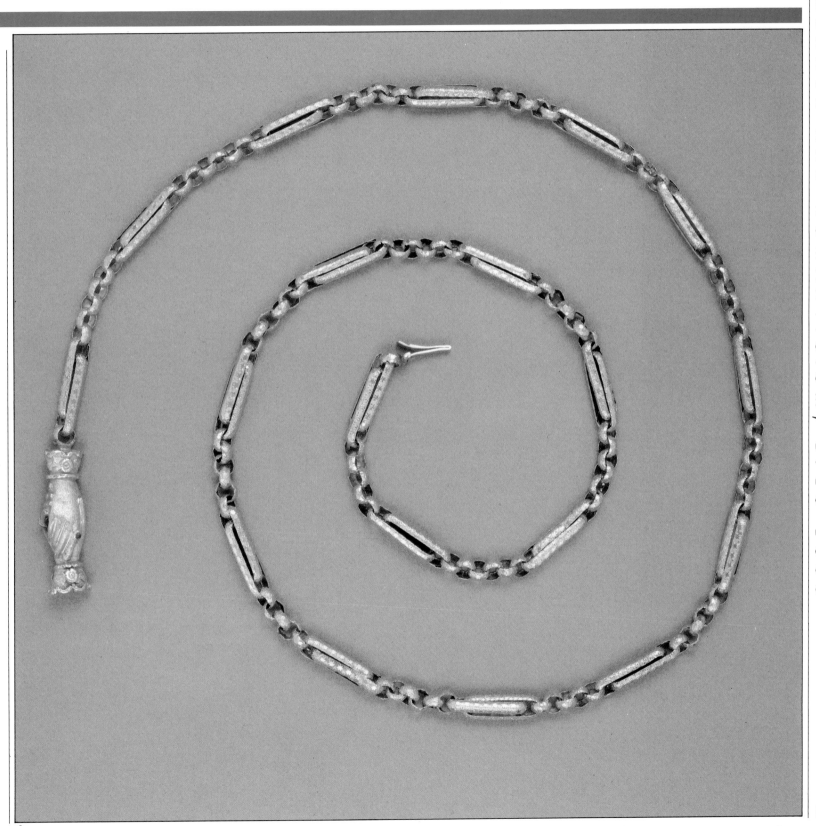

2

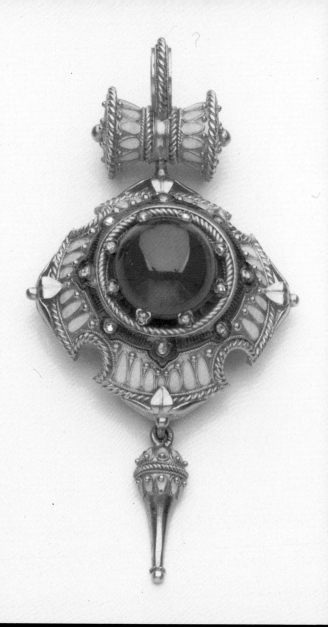

Mid-19th-century locket-back, gold pendant mounted with a garnet cabochon, surrounded by a diamond-set, white and green enameled cartouche frame,

CHAPTER FIVE

VICTORIANA AND BELLE EPOQUE

1837-1914

The art jeweler

·

The Industrial Revolution

·

Diamond refinement

·

Mourning pieces

PETER HINKS

INTRODUCTION

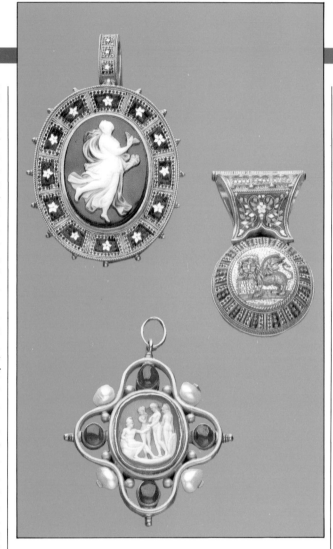

It used to be said that a Victorian jewelry fashion lasted just long enough for the lady of the house to find her maid wearing a one-and-sixpenny version of it. This is a simplification: some styles were evergreen and never out of fashion for long; others were so crazy or tasteless that they did not survive the season. Between these two extremes many fashions came and went. Certainly in this age of prosperity, and social change more people were wearing jewelry than ever before, and they were wearing more of it. Trends may be caricatured as follows: between 1840 and 1860 romantic, convoluted, grotesque, flamboyant; between 1860 and 1880 mechanistic, experimental, innovative, visual; between 1880 and 1900 subtle, elegant, witty, personal. Throughout the whole period fashions were colorful, eclectic, eccentric, sentimental, and sometimes morbid.

To some degree the 1830s represent a transition from the post-Napoleonic period. By the end of the decade grandiose parures and matched pairs of bracelets were on their way out, the frothy cannetille settings replaced by voluptuous stamped scrollwork, the pastel shades of aquamarine and pink topaz ousted by the full-blooded colors of deep garnet and turquoise. Enamel was often *en plein* – flooded all over the surface of a jewel.

By the time Victoria came to the throne in 1837 the whole mood of jewelry had changed: it was no longer neutral, a mere adjunct to the costume, but frankly romantic, a statement, a challenge even, demanding a response. An early Victorian woman of fashion wore golden serpents around her neck and wrist; a long neck chain fastened with a tiny beringed hand swayed at her waist; a jewel glimmered on her forehead; her earrings hung halfway to the shoulder. Designs were consciously elaborate, perhaps faintly perverse – rotten branches entwined like supple twigs or ribbons tangled in irresolvable knots. Gold was often "colored" or given a matte finish and smothered with engraved decoration, imparting to it the appearance of having been eaten away by time.

Jewelers began looking to the past – not learning from it as yet but borrowing from its architecture, a baroque cartouche here, a Gothic ogive there. From now on fashions in jewelry became much more sensitive to world events, and books, the theater, archeological discoveries, military campaigns, indeed anything that might be called "news," stood a strong chance of being immortalized in personal ornament.

The Romantic and nationalistic feeling that swept through Europe in the 19th century gave rise to an Indian summer of European folk art, fueled by increased earnings from the land, in which the relationship between city and peasant jewelry was never more complex. Country styles were borrowed by city jewelers and vice versa. This preoccupation with folk costume and ornament was apparent right through the century and was later to influence the Arts and Crafts Movement.

In the 1850s there was no abrupt change of direction in jewelry fashions. Gothic and particularly baroque designs were just as plentiful, although they seem to have been tighter and more formal in interpretation. Simple strap-and-buckle bracelets became popular. *Champlevé* enamel was conspicuous in white and two shades of blue; less so were the purplish almandine garnets and lemon-yellow chrysolites.

Jewelry design is related to other fashions, particularly hairstyles. When the hair covers the ears, as it did in the styles of the 1850s, there is less scope for interesting earring design, and this period saw the temporary eclipse of the earring. In the 1860s, however, the chignon appeared: the hair was now pulled back and fastened with a jeweled comb, exposing the ears. Jewelers made up for lost time, and earrings were made in a profusion of styles and designs, although always of the pendent variety. In fact, in the early part of the decade, the whole approach to jewelry changed and the emphasis shifted away from content to technique and effect. The mid-Victorian commercial

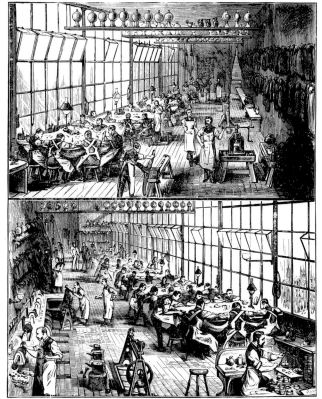

THE MANUFACTURING

GOLDSMITHS' AND SILVERSMITHS' COMPANY,

Show-Rooms: **112, REGENT-STREET, LONDON, W.** (Adjoining Stereoscopic Company.)

Supply the Public Direct at Manufacturers' Cash Prices, saving Purchasers from 25 to 50 per cent.

THE COMPANY

SUPPLY THE PUBLIC DIRECT

With Goods of their own Manufacture at a minimum profit for cash ; all intermediate profits are thereby avoided, and

THE PURCHASER
IS PLACED IN DIRECT
COMMUNICATION
WITH
THE PRODUCER.

An advantage not to be obtained at any other house or store, and effecting

A Saving varying from 25 to 50 per cent.

CATALOGUE

Containing over Five Hundred beautifully Illustrated Designs,

Gratis and Post-free to all parts of the World.

CAUTION.—The Company regret to find that many of their designs are being copied in a very inferior quality, charged at higher prices, and inserted in a similar form of advertisement, which is calculated to mislead the public.

They beg to notify that their only London retail address is 112, REGENT-STREET, W.

"A SUCCESSFUL BUSINESS."

"We know of no enterprise of recent years which has been crowned with greater success than the Goldsmiths' and Silversmiths' Company, of 112, Regent-street, who eight years ago opened their show-rooms to place the productions of their workshops direct before the public, thus saving purchasers the numerous intermediate profits which are obtained by 'middlemen' on high-class goods. Such has been the appreciation by the public that the Company have now the largest business in England, and are quite supplanting the old-fashioned houses that pride themselves upon having been established so many decades, but having utterly failed to keep pace with the times, and find it impossible to depart from their long credit system, entailing bad debts, for which cash buyers have to compensate."—Court Journal.

HIGH-CLASS JEWELLERY. The Stock of BRACELETS, BROOCHES, EARRINGS, NECKLETS, &c., is the largest and choicest in London, and contains designs of rare beauty and excellence not to be obtained elsewhere, an inspection of which is respectfully invited.

DIAMOND ORNAMENTS.—A magnificent assortment of Rings, Stars, Sprays, Flies, Necklaces, &c., composed of the finest White Diamonds, mounted in special and original designs, and sold direct to the public at merchants' cash prices.

NOVELTIES.—A succession of Novelties by the Company's own artists and designers is constantly being produced to anticipate the requirements of purchasers.

BRIDAL PRESENTS.—Special attention is devoted to the production of elegant and inexpensive novelties suitable for Bridesmaids' Presents. Original designs and estimates prepared free of charge.

WEDDING PRESENTS.

COMPLIMENTARY PRESENTS.

APPROBATION.—Selected parcels of goods forwarded to the country on approval when desired. Correspondents not being customers should send a London reference or deposit.

COUNTRY CUSTOMERS have through this means the advantage of being supplied direct from an immense London stock, containing all the latest novelties, and which are not obtainable in provincial towns.

OLD JEWELLERY, Diamonds, and Plate taken in exchange or bought for cash.

TESTIMONIALS.—The numerous recommendations with which the Goldsmiths' Company have been favoured by customers is a pleasing testimony to the excellence and durability of their manufactures.

MEDALS.—Awarded Seven Gold and Prize Medals and the Legion of Honour, the highest distinction conferred on any firm.

Jewellery and Diamond Mounting Workshops, Clerkenwell, in Direct Communication by Telephone with the Show-Rooms.
GOLDSMITHS' AND SILVERSMITHS' COMPANY, 112, REGENT-STREET.

In spite of the growth of mass production and the demands of the market, skilled craftsmanship still played a very important role in the jewelry trade. Some processes, such as setting diamonds, required a high degree of manual skill, and art jewelry was invariably made by hand. Here we see men working at benches with sheepskins slung below them to catch the "leme," or filings of previous metal. In the foreground of the upper illustration wire is being made at a drawbench, while at lower left a craftsman is polishing what appears to be a necklace. Apart from the gaslighting, a modern workshop does not look very different.

jeweler's first intention seems to have been to create a purely visual effect with patterns of light and movement, cunning arrangements of pendent drops, and reflections which subtly echoed and distorted the design. He was now prepared to explore the character of the metal without stifling it with decoration or forcing it into unnatural shapes. The lapidary took an equally experimental approach, making the stones fit the design in a way that might once have seemed cavalier. Jewelry shapes were now clean and formal: some had a disturbingly mechanistic quality like a valve or a coupling; others incorporated ideas of classical origin.

The Industrial Revolution and the Art Jeweler

It was in this period that the jewelry manufacturer tooled up for mass production. Jewels had been made by multiple production methods since ancient times, either by casting or stamping, the latter being commonplace in the first part of the 19th century. But now machines formerly powered by hand or water were turning over to gas or steam, and the pace and scope of jewelry production were vastly increased. Competition between the many firms of manufacturers was savage, resulting in a continual search for novelties and a lowering of standards in both materials and workmanship. The principal jewelry-making centers of the West where this was happening were the towns of Pforzheim in Germany, Birmingham in England, Providence in Rhode Island, and Gablonz in Bohemia.

However, while the Industrial Revolution was encroaching more and more on the world of the skilled craftsman, a new breed, the art jeweler, was emerging in Italy. Neapolitan jewelers Carlo Giuliano (1831–1895) and Giacinto Mellilo (1845–1915), and especially the Roman Fortunato Pio Castellani (1794–1865), created jewels of small intrinsic value but extraordinary beauty which established the Greek and Etruscan style as the most influential of the period. Some of their jewels were precise copies of Greek or Etruscan originals; others were more in the nature of pastiches. These jewelers were genuinely trying to learn from the past, using it as a repository of ideas and knowledge rather than a box of design tricks.

INTRODUCTION

Castellani, the leading light in this revivalist movement, realized that the ancient Greeks and Etruscans could do things that were beyond his skill and set about trying to rediscover their secrets. The Giuliano family, who came to work in London, moved toward the Italian Renaissance as a source of inspiration, and their achievement was to express the spirit of the late 19th century in its eloquent language.

But perhaps more important than the jewels made by the Italians was the change in attitude which they

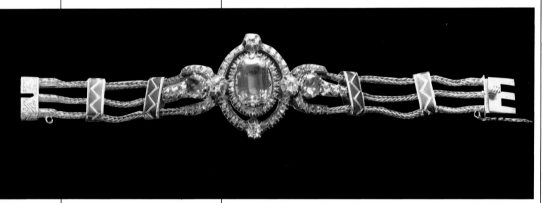

A gold, sapphire, diamond, and enamel bracelet.

heralded. We are beginning to see the first stirrings of an industrial counter-revolution: from 1860 onward there was a growing reaction against the machine, its effects on people's lives, and the soulless quality of the things it produced. Disillusioned with much of what was on offer, many women of the intelligentsia simply got off the fashion merry-go-round and either wore no jewelry at all or else went ethnic with peasant jewelry. Others patronized the art jewelers like Giuliano and Castellani, who thought of their work as a vocation rather than a trade.

In Paris at this time there was a renaissance in the art of enameling, and in the second half of the century techniques that had long fallen into disuse were successfully revived. The exquisite *plique à jour* was rediscovered, and Riffaut (1832–1872) made a series of jewels in this magical technique for Frédéric Boucheron, the great impresario of Parisian jewelry. His experiments were of great importance to Lalique and the Art Nouveau jewelers of the 1890s. René Lalique himself (1860–1945) also made jewels in *basse taille.* Lucien Falize traveled to Japan, newly opened to the West, to learn the art of cloisonné. Without exception, all of the great techniques of enameling on metal were thriving in the French capital at this time

The Diamond Workers

In the highly specialized jewelry business the workers in diamonds, both cutters and setters, were and are distinct from the rest of the trade. In this field

there was nothing to be learned from the past, and new ground was being broken all the time. Diamonds certainly became more plentiful in the 19th century. In the 18th and early 19th centuries Brazil was the primary producer, reaching a peak in the mid-1800s after the discovery of the Bahia fields in 1844. Diamond jewelry at this time was very magnificent in designs of scrolls, ribbons and, above all, flowers.

Since the 18th century jewelers had been trying to imitate flowers and plants in precious metals and diamonds. As their techniques improved the results became less stylized and more naturalistic. They had already learned how to mount a flower *en tremblant* on a spiral spring so that it quivered with the wearer's movements. Settings became lighter and less obtrusive. The naturalistic style reached its apotheosis in the work of a jeweler working in Paris. Oliver Massin (born 1829, retired 1892) invented a method of making the plant stem in tubular sections so that it could be threaded on a length of spring steel, a more natural way of achieving the *tremblant* effect. For the diamond setter the introduction of platinum at the end of the 19th century meant an important change. The great mechanical strength of platinum now enabled him to make mounts that were almost invisible once the stones were set. Another change in the diamonds world was brought about by the arrival of stones from South Africa in 1870. Until then brilliants had been left square and deep, conforming to the shape of the natural crystal, but now that there was such a plentiful supply of diamonds from the Cape the gem could be cut round and shallow, which was extravagant of material but made for a brighter stone.

The diamond jewelry made between the closing years of the 19th century and the outbreak of the First World War has probably never been matched in any period. There was a distinctive 18th-century flavor about many of these jewels, and 18th-century styles, with their rococo scrolls and latticed backgrounds were in evidence. Just as popular were the Victorian perennials – stars, Maltese crosses, and crescents – which were being advertised for sale by jewelers at least as late as 1906.

In the 19th century, where the explorer went, the prospector followed, leading to discoveries of precious minerals, some of them new to science. The enchanting green demantoid garnet was unknown until the 1860s, when specimens were found in Siberia. Crocidolite, or tiger's eye, a golden-brown gem with a satiny sheen, was discovered in large deposits in South West Africa. Black opal was found on Lightning Ridge, Queensland; superb sapphires, in Kashmir – until then they had been used as gunflints. The Burmese ruby mines were exploited commercially. Gold was discovered in California, Australia, and South Africa. As a result of these discoveries, we are left now with large quantities of 19th-century jewelry: the new abundance of raw materials not only kept the workshops well supplied but also removed much of the need to melt down old jewels to make new.

Mourning Jewelry

Certain kinds of Victorian jewelry reflected the sentimentality of the age. Many jewels were fitted with tiny crystal compartments to contain locks of hair, and sentimental inscriptions abound. "Mizpah" is a fairly common one and signifies, "The Lord watch between me and thee when we are absent one from another." An anchor, a cross, and a heart on a jewel represent the virtues of Faith, Hope, and Charity. The practice of wearing mourning jewelry was already well established, and in the 1840s the enameled cartouches set with crystal hair compartments and rings with forget-me-nots and pearls for tears, charming jewels in their own right, still retained something of the wistful quality of mourning jewelry of the late 18th century. As time went on and mourning rituals became more prescribed and demanding, the market for this jewelry increased until its manufacture assumed the proportions of an industry.

Mourning jewelry was made in a variety of materials which could be of "any color so long as it was black": enamel, jet, onyx, glass, Berlin cast iron, papier mâché, vulcanite (an early form of plastic), and petrified oak from the Irish bogs. Most included a lock of the dead person's hair preserved under a little window and a brief epitaph with the appropriate names and dates. Later designs were formal and chilly, expressing awfulness and finality rather than sadness and regret. The dour and dreadful figure of Victoria grieving for her lost Albert had a lot to answer for, but as her influence waned in the more relaxed atmosphere of the Belle Epoque, mourning jewelry was less in evidence.

Belle Epoque

The influence of King Edward VII and his enchanting Danish bride Alexandra was felt long before they came to the throne. They encouraged fashions that were exuberant but disciplined, gay but not wanton. Shapes became more fluent, colors softer, under the influence of Art Nouveau. Colored stones of every kind were worn, especially the more exotic varieties – alexandrite, demantoid garnet, and cat's eye. The leek-green peridot was said to be the favorite stone of the Prince of Wales. Alexandra was seen to like mauve, so amethysts were fashionable. But without doubt it was the diamond and the pearl that held pride of place. Pearls were worn either as a long *sautoir* or close to the throat in several short strings as a *collier de chien*; curiously shaped baroque pearls from the Mississippi freshwater mussel were hung as pendants from many semiprecious jewels.

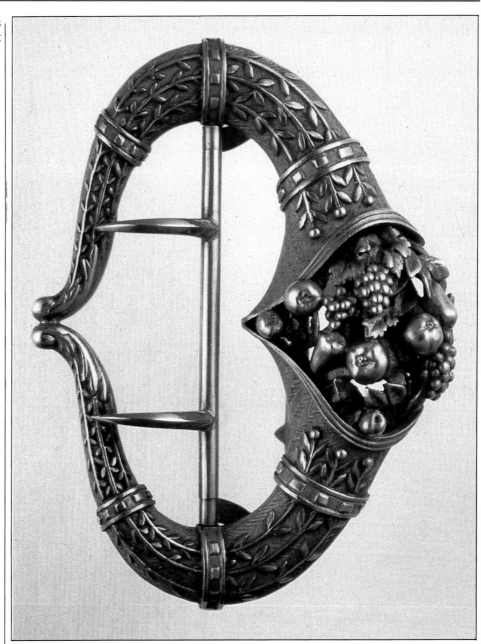

A gold and enamel buckle designed by Chardon and made by Le Turcq for Boucheron in 1903.

INFLUENCES

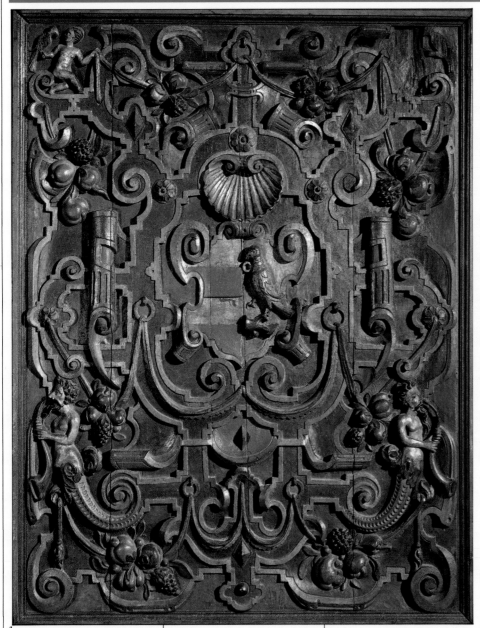

1

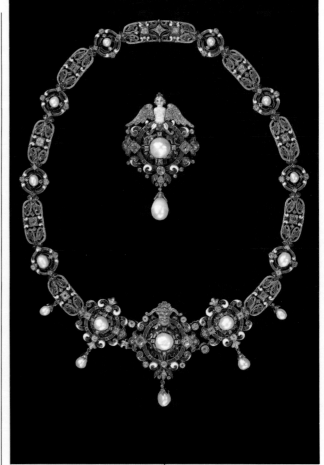

2

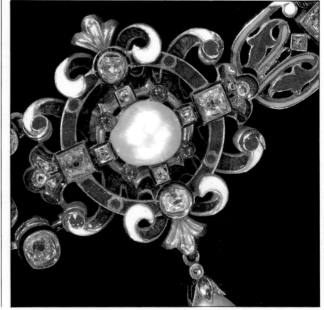

The Renaissance may be counted, along with Gothic and Classical Greek styles, among the most important historical influences to shape Victorian jewelry fashions. It appeared in different interpretations; motifs were often lifted from architecture – caryatids, cartouches, and strapwork – and composed in ornaments which, although very effective, bore no resemblance to Renaissance jewelry. The intricate strapwork and figures in this early 17th-century oak panel (**1**), carved in relief, painted, and gilded, are echoed in a lavishly executed necklace and brooch (**2**), c. 1860. Fashioned in the French Neo-Renaissance style by Rodolphi, a Danish jeweler working in Paris in the middle of the 19th century, it is in enameled gold set with emeralds, rubies, diamonds, and hung with pearls. The Renaissance motifs are repeated in the putto and satyr which crown both the brooch and the necklace, a detail of which is shown at right.

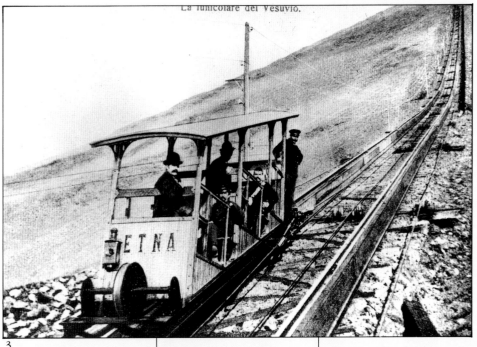

3

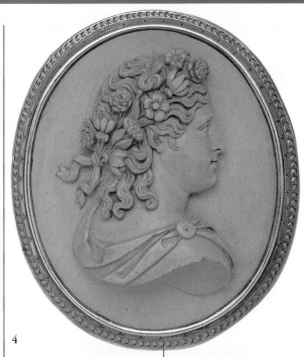

4

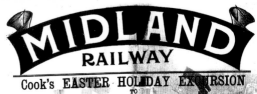

6

MIDLAND RAILWAY

Cook's EASTER HOLIDAY EXCURSION
TO
SCOTLAND.

ON THURSDAY, APRIL 9TH
FOR 5 or 8 DAYS,

From BRISTOL, Clifton Down, Redland, Montpelier, BATH, Gloucester, Cheltenham, Worcester, Malvern, Evesham, Alcester, and Redditch (to certain Stations), BIRMINGHAM, WOLVERHAMPTON, WALSALL, Tamworth, Burton, and DERBY, to

EDINBURGH, GLASGOW
CARLISLE, DUMFRIES, CASTLE DOUGLAS,
Kirkcudbright, Greenock, Ayr
KILMARNOCK, STIRLING, PERTH,
DUNDEE, ARBROATH, FORFAR, BRECHIN,
MONTROSE, STONEHAVEN,
ABERDEEN, INVERNESS, &c.

THIRD CLASS RETURN TICKETS
Will also be issued by these trains, to return any day within 16 Days from date of issue.

For Times, Fares, Conditions, etc. see Small Bills.

For Tickets and further particulars of above, and of Tourist and Excursion Arrangements in SCOTLAND, see Programmes to be obtained at the Booking Offices of the MIDLAND RAILWAY COMPANY, or at the Offices of

Thos. Cook & Son,

Originators of the European Excursion and Tourist System—Established 1841.

JOHN MATHIESON, General Manager.

Thos. Cook & Son, Printers, London and Birmingham.

5

Wherever the Victorian tourist went in search of ruins or mountains, jewelers busied themselves making souvenirs. In Italy, the romantic traveler scaled Vesuvius on the funicular railway (3) and brought back cameos carved from Vesuvian lava, (this one, 4, set in gold, c. 1850-80),

mosaics from Rome and Florence, and coral from Naples and Genoa. Thomas Cook (5) exploited the fashion set by the Queen for everything Scottish, and astute Scots devised a variety of pieces to tempt the traveler: jewels set with grouse claws, granite, freshwater pearls, and above all, polished

agates and jaspers from the surrounding hills, and known as Scotch pebble jewelry. The Scotch pebble bracelet and brooches (6) are set in silver, the central one in the shape of a Scottish dirk.

THE EARLY YEARS

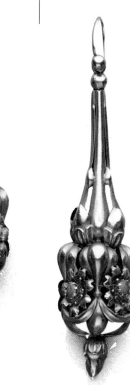
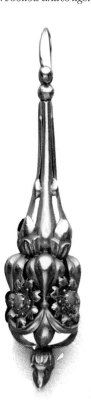

*These gold and turquoise pendant earrings (**1**) of c. 1840 are built up from elements of stamped sheet metal. Although large, the earrings are hollow and so light in weight.*

1

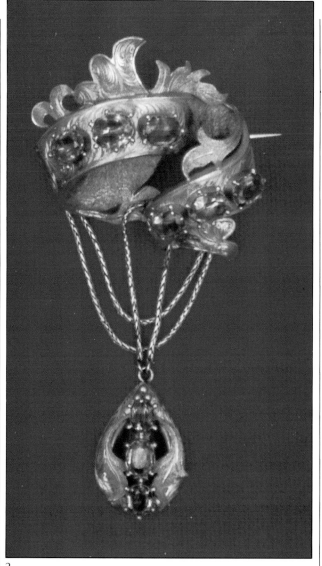

2

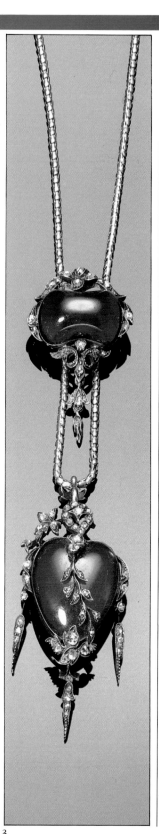

*The rococo design and elaborately festooned chains of this gold and pink topaz brooch (**2**) are typically mid-19th century, as is the top of the carbuncle (a type of garnet) and diamond pendant (**3**) (c. 1855), which forms a coulant designed to slide freely on the tubular chain. The buxom curves and plushy color of the carbuncles are set off by the sparkle and delicacy of the diamond foliage, which also helps to hold the two big cabochons in place. The oatgrain-shaped diamond drops are characteristic of the period.*

3

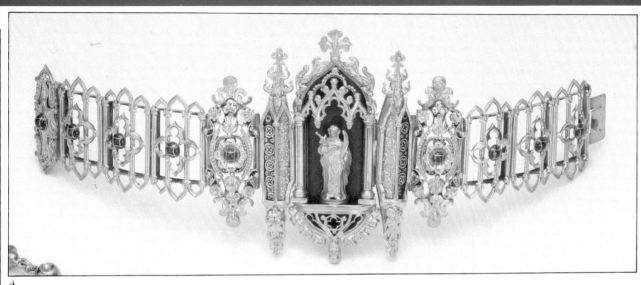

A gold and enamel bracelet based on Gothic architecture, probably French, c. 1845 (4).

4

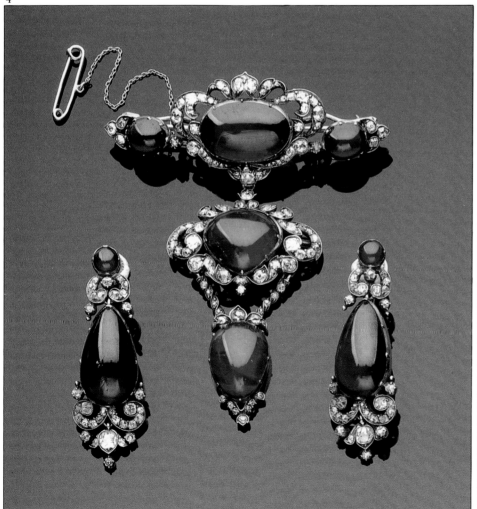

6

5

The scrollwork on the gold and turquoise cartouche-shaped brooch (5) contrasts well with the matte ground. In the mid-19th century brooches tended to be designed along the horizontal axis. This is a machine-made piece of good quality, c. 1840 In the garnet and diamond demi-parure (6) the substantial pavé-set diamond scrollwork is kept clear of the garnets, which are held in place with a "cut-down" setting, that is a rim of gold filed to a bevel but with small points of metal left to buttress it. The design, and engineering, and the presence of a pair of earrings indicate a date in the 1840s.

THE ART JEWELER

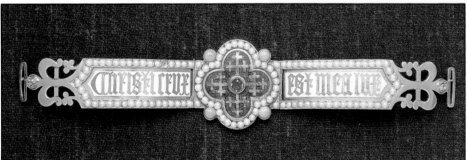

This necklace and pair of matching pendants (**1**) are possibly from a diadem. Finely decorated with filigree and granulation, the pendants are embossed with Thetis riding a sea monster and carrying the armor of Achilles. These jewels were made by Castellani in around 1870, after Greek originals excavated at Kul Oba, in southern Russia, in 1864.

1

2

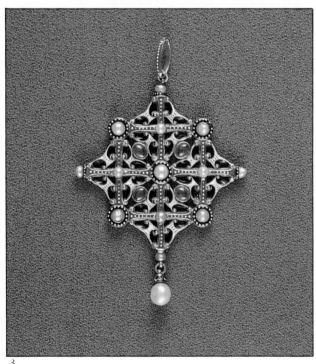

The headband in gold and champlevé enamel set with a ruby and turquoises (**2**) was designed by A. W. N. Pugin (1812–52) in the Gothic style and made by John Hardman and Co. in 1848. Pugin was the first designer to reject the machine and advocate a return to hand craftsmanship and therefore foreshadowed the Arts and Crafts movement. Regrettably he designed very little jewelry.

A gold, cabochon ruby, and pearl pendant (**3**) by Giuliano in their own distinctive interpretation of the Renaissance style. The Giuliano family often used black and white enamel in this way, to tone down rather than enhance the color-scheme of a jewel.

3

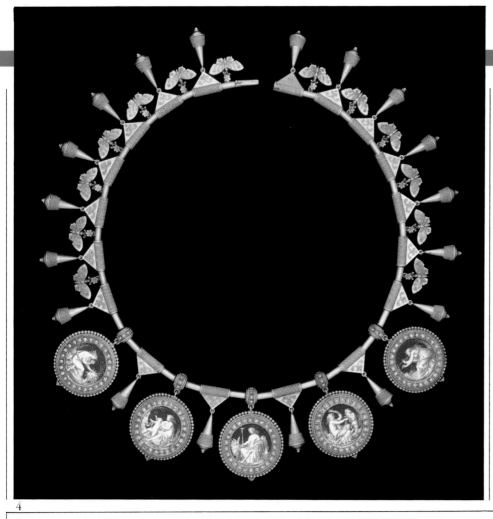

This necklace of gold and diamonds (4) is set with painted enamels of nymphs and cupids in "Pompeian" style and is by Eugène Fontenay (1823–87), the leading exponent in France of the Greek Revivalist style: the drop-shaped pendants and butterflies have apparently been borrowed from Greek and Etruscan jewelry.

4

BOUCHERON

Frédéric Boucheron opened his first shop in Paris, in the Place du Palais Royal, in 1858. From the outset he showed an extraordinary intuitive response to the tastes and fashions of his time. There was scarcely a style or a new technique in which he was not intimately concerned, if he was not its actual instigator. He was showing *plique à jour* enamel, which years later was to become synonymous with Art Nouveau, at the Paris Exhibition of 1867, while Lalique was still a child. The Mogul emperors retained lapidaries skilled enough to engrave diamond, the hardest substance known – so did Boucheron. Like Benvenuto Cellini he made jewels of chiseled steel.

Boucheron was a keen observer of nature and brought something greater than realism to the translation of living plants into jewels, selecting not merely the conventional roses and marigolds, but hedgerow thistles and spectacular twigs of plane tree leaves. His jewelry typified everything the American traveling millionaire was looking for in late 19th-century Europe. It was daring, original, chic, and of superb quality in both materials and workmanship. The firm moved to the Place Vendôme in 1893. A branch was opened in Moscow in 1902, but Frédéric did not live to see the firm established in London and New York in the following year. He was succeeded by his son Louis.

A pair of hair ornaments in plique à jour *enamel, diamonds, and pearls, made by Riffault, c. 1870, for Boucheron.*

5

MID-CENTURY WORK

This 1870s bracelet of colored golds (**1**) is inlaid in a diapered pattern and set with turquoise. Checkered patterns and variations on them were popular after London's Great Exhibition of 1852. The smooth finish and massive appearance are typically mid-Victorian. The gold and Florentine mosaic brooch (**2**) has a mosaic inlay of white shell and malachite on a ground of black marble and dates from c. 1860.

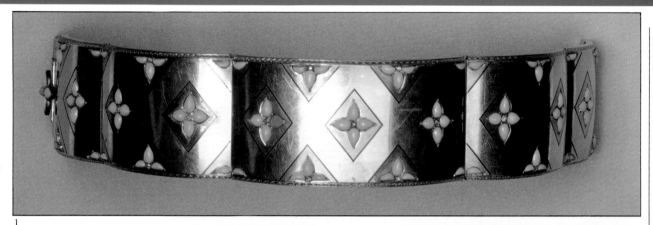

1

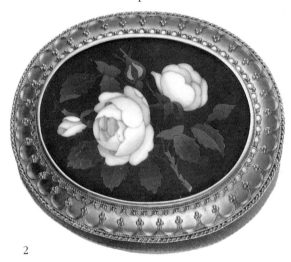

2

(**3**) At the top, a gold, turquoise, enamel, and half-pearl demi-parure of 1870. The necklace, with its festoons of "brazilian" chain and fringed pendants, illustrates a basic theme which appeared in numerous variations, often with a classical Greek flavor, throughout the 1860s and after. The circular form of the brooch is also typical, as is the broad hinged bracelet. To the left is a gold and turquoise padlock. Lock and key jewels are eternal and universal; for example, in the Far East they are worn to preserve life by locking in the soul while in the West they are tokens of love. This example was probably a bracelet fastening. Below, a gold and carbuncle bracelet of 1860 in a very simple Gothic design; and bottom, a gold necklace in classical Greek style from the last 30 years of the 19th century. The small holes pierced in the hollow drops are not purely decorative, but also served to vent expanding gases when they were being soldered.

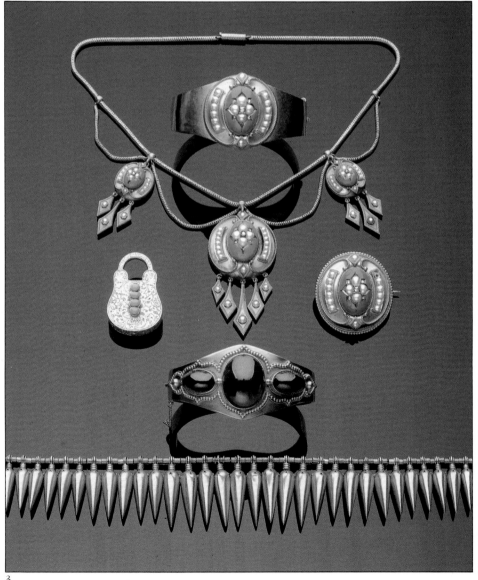

3

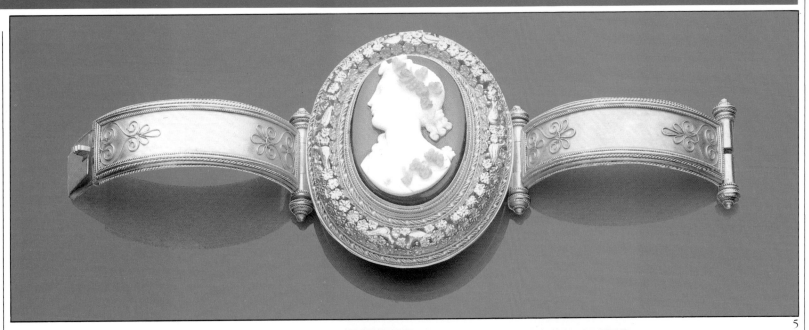

5

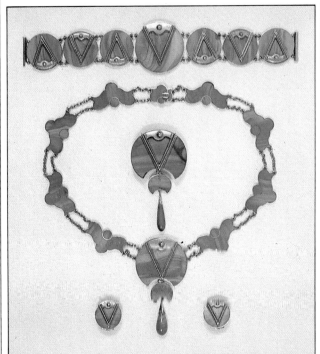

4

The stones of the gold and
malachite parure (**4**) are cut in
unconventional shapes and
applied with a mechanistic
quadrant and rivet-head design.

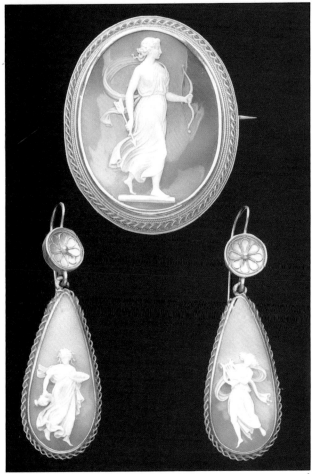

A cameo bracelet of c. 1880 made
of gold and sardonyx (**5**).
Sardonyx is a type of agate formed
in alternate layers of flesh pink
and white. To cut a cameo the
stone is oriented so that the layers
run parallel to the surface. The
design is cut in the white so that the
flesh-colored background is
exposed. In this case the stone has
been worked in three layers and is
set in a border of flowers and
doves. In the gold and shell cameo
demi-parure (**6**) the cameos have
been cut from a conch shell, which
resembles sardonyx in that it has a
stratified structure with a pale
outer layer and a flesh-colored
lining. Being softer than sardonyx,
it is easier to work, which makes it
less durable, but it is cheaper. The
back of a sardonyx usually reveals
the concavity of a sea shell. Jewels
of the design illustrated have been
made for the tourist trade from
1860 to the present.

6

97

MOURNING JEWELRY

The mount of this gold mourning locket (**1**) set with black onyx applied with a rose diamond and freshwater pearl star, is engraved and decorated with champlevé enamel.

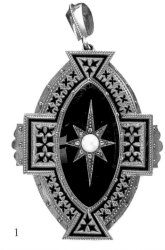

1

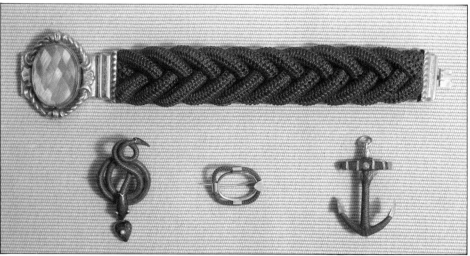

2

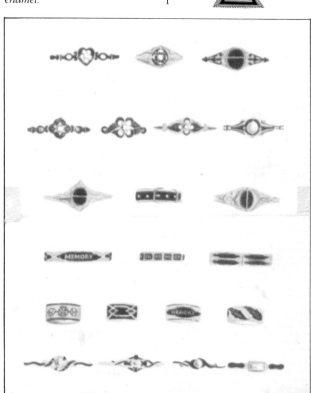

3

These designs for mourning rings by John Brogden (**3**) were taken from an album of designs found recently in the jeweler's archive.

A mid 19th-century bracelet of braided hair, (**2**) the clasp set with a hair compartment. The gold mounts have been stamped out by machine. Below, the gold and hair brooch representing an anchor may have signified that the person commemorated was a seafarer, or may have been used as a symbol of the Christian faith. To its left, a gold, enamel, and hair brooch represents a snake with a heart pendent from its jaws, a favored early Victorian motif.

The fringe of chain on the gold and black-enamel mourning brooch (**4**) is often seen in jewels of the 1860s. The reverse is dated 1866.

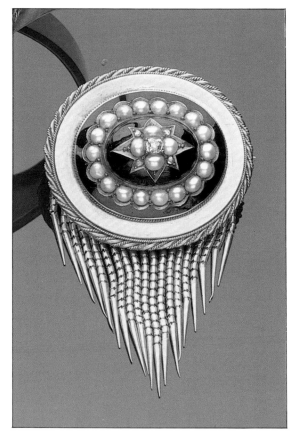

4

MACHINE-MADE JEWELRY

The garnet necklace (**1**) was made in Gablonz, Bohemia, in the late 19th century. This cheap and effective jewelry was exported all over Europe. The locally mined stones were often but by children and set in very low carat gold.

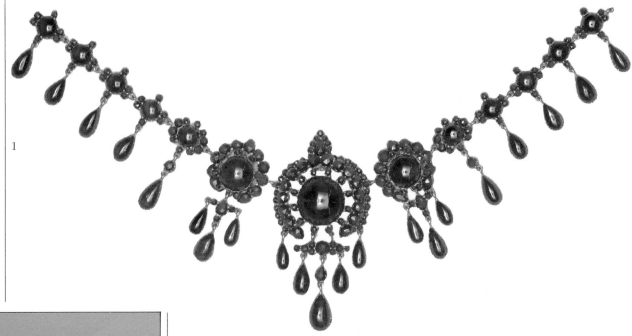

1

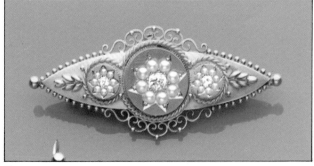

2

The front and back of the late 19th-century brooch (**2**) would have been stamped out separately and soldered together. The borders and brooch fitting would be added at this stage and the stones set last of all.

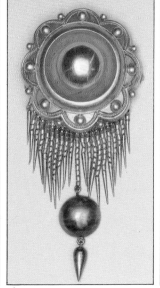

4

3

Making the dies for a machine-made jewel is the most expensive part of the process. However, few would be needed to produce this simple bracelet (**3**) which was made in the mid-19th century, probably in central Europe, and relatively little handwork would be required to finish it. This good quality gold brooch (**4**) was made in the 1860s, probably in England, the birthplace of the Industrial Revolution, where a huge amount of jewelry was produced in small backstreet workshops. The incomplete article would be passed from one workshop to another for each stage of the manufacturing process.

NOVELTIES

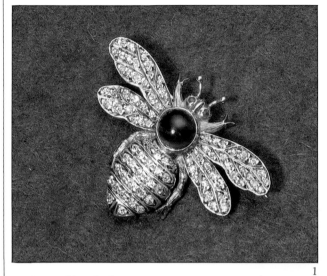

1

A demantoid garnet and diamond bird brooch (**2**). Demantoid garnets were first discovered in Siberia in the Ural Mountains in 1860. Jewels set with these stones, which rival the diamond in fire and the peridot in color, were very fashionable in late Victorian and Edwardian times.

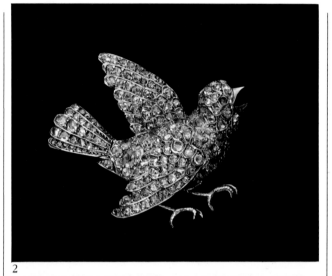

2

The design of this cabochon amethyst and diamond bumble-bee brooch (**1**) of c. 1890 probably had its origin in the Second Empire, the bee was an emblem of the House of Bonaparte. Winged insects – gadflies, dragonflies, butterflies, even houseflies – were very popular in jewelry from 1860.

The carved carbuncle, emerald, and rose-diamond beetle brooch (**3**) dates from c. 1865. Large and grotesque beetle brooches are usually of French origin.

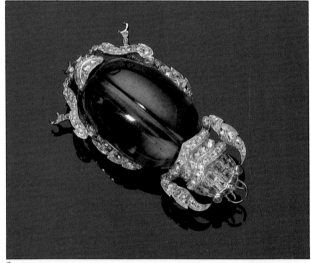

3

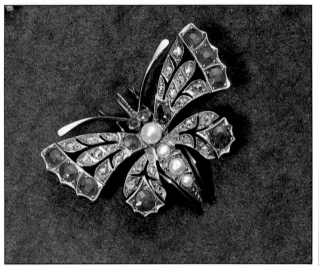

4

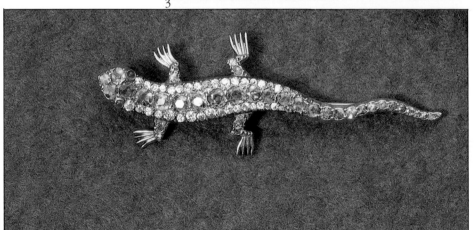

5

Butterfly brooches of this type (**4**) were manufactured in large numbers at the turn of the century. This is an inexpensive little jewel set with rose diamonds and colored stones. Small brooches were worn several at a time, and in 1907 they helped to anchor the masses of lace which cascaded down the corsage.

A demantoid garnet and diamond lizard brooch (**5**). Both frog and lizard brooches set with these gems were popular around 1900. The frog was a universal symbol of love, while the natural color of the lizard makes it an ideal vehicle for the fashionable demantoid garnet.

The decoration of this enamel and half-pearl heart pendant (**6**), made c. 1900, is derived from the 18th century, although in the original enamel would probably have been blue rather than green. The brooch (**7**) representing a "merrythought" or wishbone, uses the cockerel motif, following the success of Emile Rostand's comedy Chanticleer. *It is also the national emblem of France. The cock wards off bad luck because its cry scares away the evil forces of the night.*

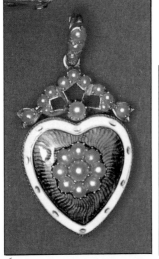

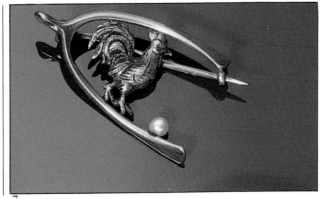

6

7

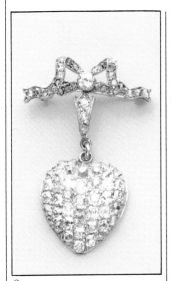

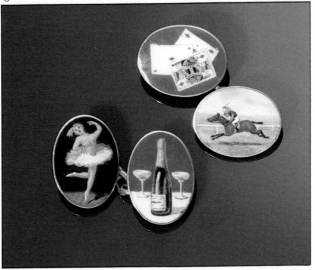

8

9

10

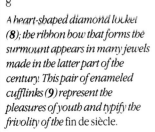

A heart-shaped diamond locket (**8**); the ribbon bow that forms the surmount appears in many jewels made in the latter part of the century. This pair of enameled cufflinks (**9**) represent the pleasures of youth and typify the frivolity of the fin de siècle.

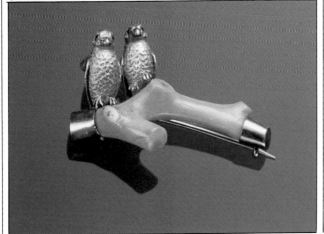

11

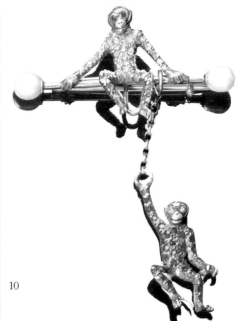

A ruby and diamond monkey brooch (**10**) of c. 1880. Popular literature and art of the late 19th and early 20th centuries were preoccupied with the notion of man's evolution through the ages.

A gold brooch (**11**) representing a pair of lovebirds perched on a coral branch dating from the last quarter of the 19th century.

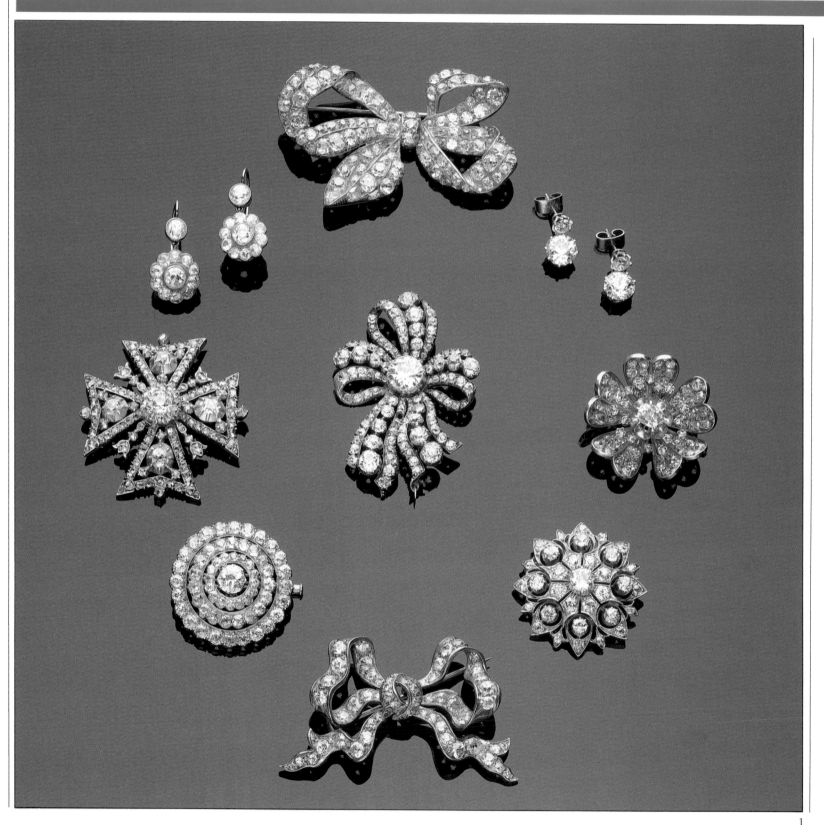

(**1**) The naturalism of the three ribbon-bow brooches and the Alexandra rose is typical of the Belle Epoque and in vivid contrast with the more formal Victorian star, cross, and target designs. All, however, are long-standing favorites, returning to fashion time and again in one form or another. There would be little difference between this very English Maltese cross and one made three-quarters of a century earlier.

The diamond aigrette (**3**) was designed to be worn in the hair with an osprey – a plume of egret feathers. This style was introduced in the 1890s but persisted in one form or another until well after the First World War. Winged hair ornaments are said to have been popularized by Boucheron, and this was also a time when Western man was obsessed with the idea of flight.

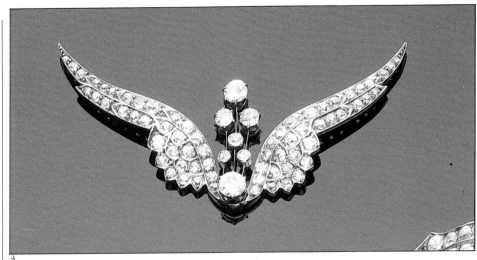

3

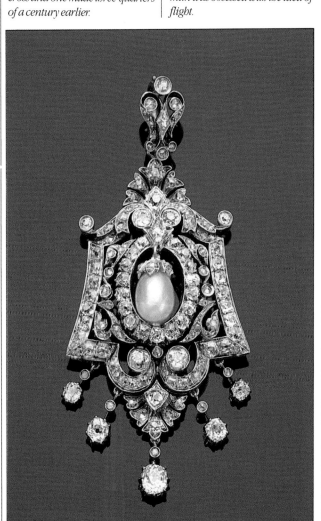

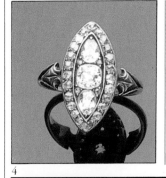

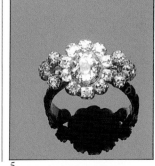

4

5

The gold and diamond scrollwork of this pearl and diamond pendant (**2**), enclosed in a somewhat architectural border, hint at a Continental rather than an English origin and suggest a date in the last quarter of the 19th century.

In the years before the First World War, rings were worn in considerable numbers, sometimes one or more on each finger. This boat-shaped marquise ring (**4**) is typical of the period, and (**5**) also dates from this time.

Swags, garlands, and ribbon bows are characteristic of the Belle Epoque. As the style moved on into the 20th century designs became more stylized; this charming corsage ornament (**6**) dates from just before the First World War.

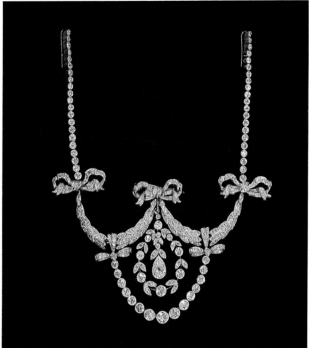

2

6

DIAMONDS

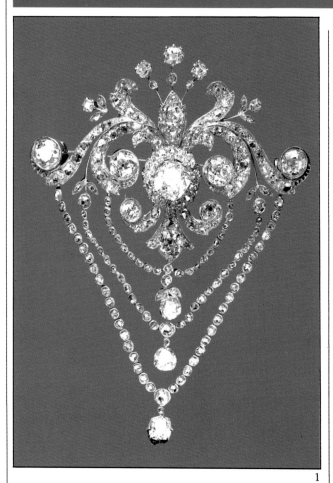

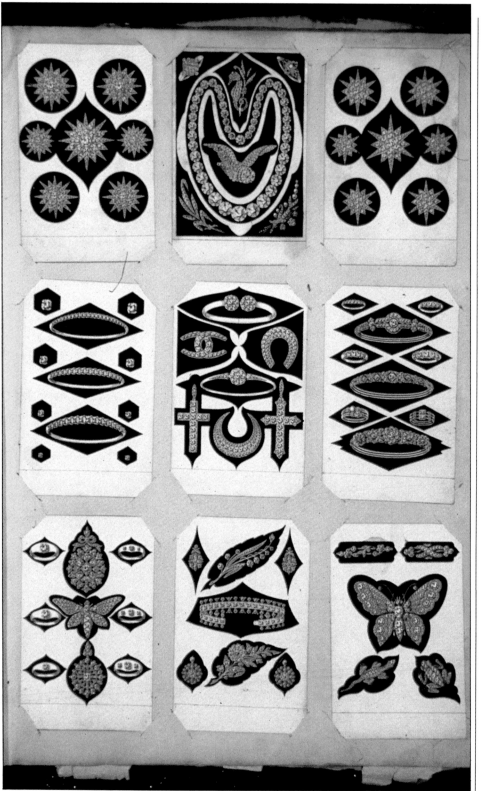

This diamond stomacher brooch (*1*) has a scroll design sprigged with foliage and is surmounted by a spray of collet-set diamonds mounted on knife wires; it dates from the last quarter of the 19th century.

Designs for diamond jewelry by Watherston and Brogden (*2*). The stars (top left and right) are designed to be worn either singly as suites of brooches or screwed on to a frame as a tiara. The sea-horse brooch (top center) is very uncommon, but diamond owls are met with from time to time. The rest – the rivière necklace, the crosses, half-hoop bracelets, butterfly brooches, flower sprays, horseshoes, etc – are all representative of a first-class late Victorian London jeweler's stock-in-trade.

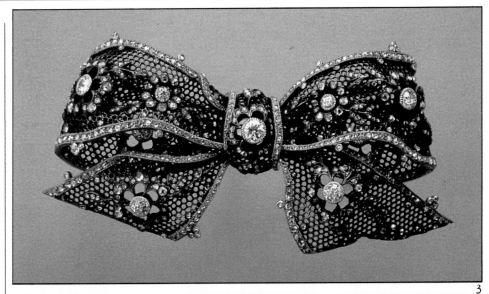

The idea of the bow brooch arises directly out of the costume and blends very closely with it when worn. This illustration (3) shows a corsage ornament in which the connection is carried to its logical conclusion. The lace of the bow is of blackened platinum sprigged with diamond flowers and with an edging of gold and diamonds. This construction is not only decorative but very light in wear. Made by Lefort for Boucheron in 1908.

3

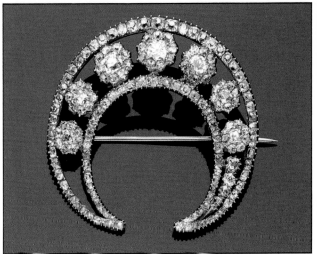

4

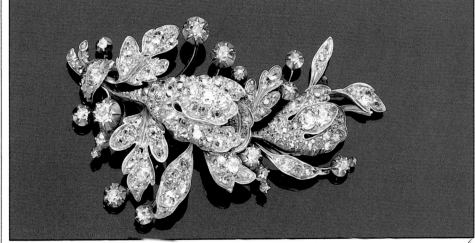

6

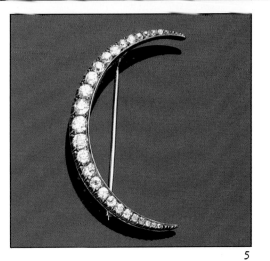

5

The crescent is perhaps the oldest of jewel designs. This simple theme exists in many variants, two of which are illustrated (4 and 5). Most of those made in the last quarter of the 19th century are primarily brooches, but were provided with a pronged fitting which allowed them also to be worn in the hair "à la Diane." This diamond spray brooch is a design of wild anemones (6) from the mid-19th century.

BELLE EPOQUE

A peridot and diamond pendant brooch (**1**) in a design of garlanded ribbons and flowers, c.1890. The leek-green peridot was said to have been the favorite stone of Edward, Prince of Wales. The quiet tints and subtle effects of semi-precious stones like aquamarine, cat's eye, alexandrite, moonstone, and the Australian and Mexican opal were very appropriate to the light, open designs of this time. Half-hoop bracelet designs proliferated from 1870 onward. The simple theme of a hinged and clasped hoop, with the decoration confined to the front, lent itself to many variations, some quite elaborate. The illustration (**2**) shows cluster, foliate and entrelac de rubans designs. The crossover, fourth from the left, was very popular.

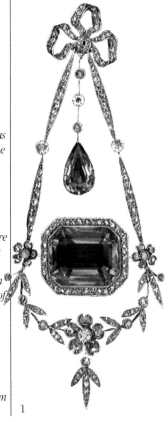

1

QUEEN ALEXANDRA

The combined influence of Edward VII and his beautiful Danish bride Alexandra was felt long before the couple came to the throne. Two jewelry styles co existed at that time: Victorian, which was formal and impressive, and Edwardian, which had a more cosmopolitan flavor. Alexandra herself was a woman of simple tastes, content to wear no ornament other than a single rose in the daytime. State occasions required her to dress for the part, however, and she did so with dignity and flair. Around her neck she customarily wore a close-fitting *collier de chien*, a fashion she is said to have adopted to conceal a small scar on her throat.

She favored a tiara in the imperial Russian style, the design of which was based on a peasant head dress, the *kokoshnik*. When Alexandra came to the throne jewelry was worn more creatively to suit the age and looks of the wearer: here she wears the tiara perched on top of a mass of curls. This new freedom had its limits. At dinner Edward was once heard to say to a lady guest, "The Princess has taken the trouble to wear a tiara-why haven't you?"

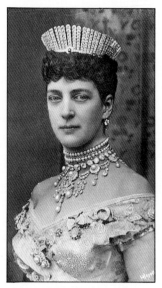

Queen Alexandra dressed for a state occasion.

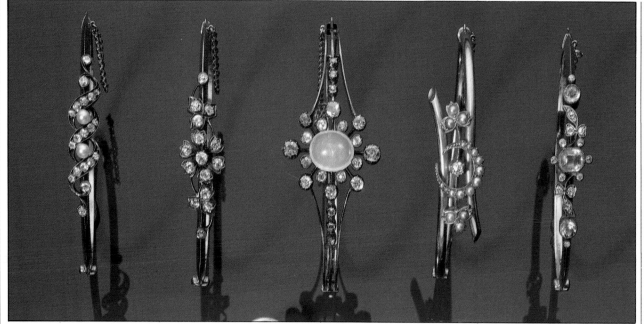

A necklace (**3**) reputed to have once belonged to Queen Alexandra. The hexagonal outlines of the amethysts blend more readily with the diamond scrollwork than would more conventional circular shapes. This regal jewel is saved from being overwhelming by the pendant garlands and undulating scrollwork which also give it an 18th-century flavor. The Queen often wore amethysts, said to be her favorite stones.

A pearl and diamond necklace dating from the last half of the 19th century. This jewel may also be adapted for wear as a tiara.

A late 19th-century diamond crescent brooch.

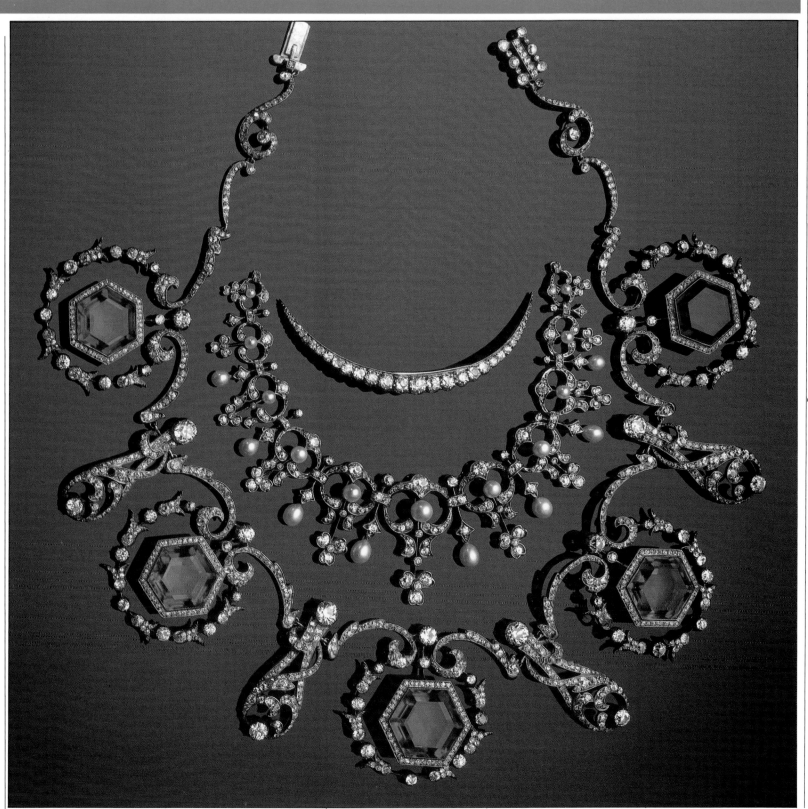

3

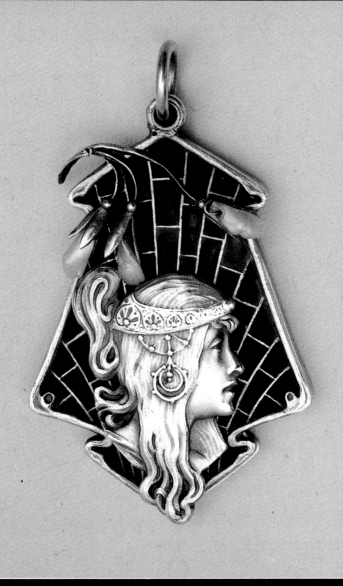

Pendant of silver-gilt and plique à jour enamel with three baroque pearl blossoms. German or Austrian, c. 1900-10.

CHAPTER · SIX
JEWELRY FOR AESTHETES

1875-1919

INTRODUCTION

Maison Vever, one of Paris's best-known joailliers in the Art Nouveau period, produced the stunning pendant-brooch and necklace. The works of the brothers Paul and Henri Vever were more restrained and controlled than those of their admired contemporary René Lalique, but nonetheless bore similar motifs and were as expertly executed. Of enameled gold, diamonds, and sapphires, the pendant features two facing peacocks, their feet centered on a large pearl. The peacock was a popular Art Nouveau subject, its showy plumage often represented in jewelry, glass, fabric, etc.

The quarter-century or so leading up to the year 1900 embraced on the one hand the waning of the Victorian era and on the other the onset of the modern age. The Industrial Revolution rumbled on; electricity and photography were nascent sciences; innovative technologies were bursting upon an advancing Western world – and the first fine art to be called "modern" (by later art historians) was being created by Manet, Cézanne, Monet, and their contemporaries.

In the decorative arts, too, signs of a new age were beginning to reveal themselves, in techniques, materials, themes, influences, and purpose, and jewelry was one of the most visible and exciting of the plastic arts to display these signs in, appropriately enough, the vocabulary of the turn-of-the-century Art Nouveau ("New Art") style. Art Nouveau was a French design movement characterized by whiplash curves, references to nature, and virtuoso techniques; and nowhere was this better seen than in goldsmiths' work, notably the jewels of Reńe Lalique, the Maison Vever, and Georges Fouquet. Gallic Art Nouveau made waves throughout all of Europe and the Americas, but so too did the Jugendstil ("Young Style") jewels of Germany, the decidedly modernist works of Austria's Wiener Werkstätte, and the vast related output of American and other European designers, some anonymous, others well known. Designers of the hand-crafted and mass-produced jewelry of Great Britain, including that of Liberty & Co. and the Glasgow School, shared an aesthetic, a design philosophy, and working methods of the German and Austrian jewelers, and were linked by their use of materials.

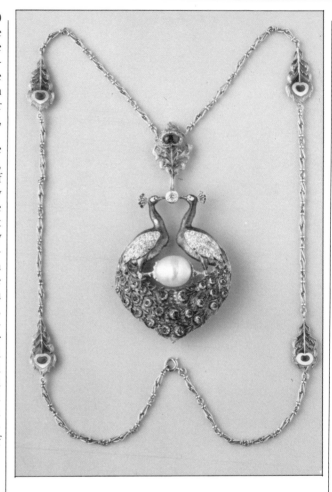

The Arts and Crafts Designers

The Arts and Crafts Movement is generally considered as one which looked back, rather than ahead, for its inspiration and guiding principles. The movement, whose leading exponents were the critic John Ruskin and the multi-talented designer–writer–activist William Morris, was essentially a reaction against the encroaching modern age, against the squalor and ills that were perceived to have been brought on by industrialization, against the shoddy, machine-made products that were being spewed forth. Arts and Crafts designs – interiors, architecture, furniture, books, metalwork, and jewelry – signaled a romantic, though not rigid, return to earlier, purer aesthetics and techniques; their creators took their inspiration largely from what they viewed as the simple, unsullied Middle Ages – its cathedrals, furnishings, even costumes, and perhaps, most significantly, its workers' guilds and their guiding rules and methods.

The finest Arts and Crafts pieces are one-off, appreciated not for their value or their weight, but for their design, their color, their workmanship. Unlike most French or Belgian Art Nouveau pieces, the Arts and Crafts designs tended to be simple, even somewhat primitive, figural or floral motifs, or more complex, interlaced (*entrelac*) or knotted patterns of Celtic inspiration. This latter type of design was best shown off on myriad belt or waist buckles and clasps by designers like Oliver Baker, Archibald Knox, Kate Fisher, Kate Allen, and Edgar Simpson (many of them sold at Liberty). For the stone-set pieces – which included brooches, pendants, bracelets, necklaces, hatpins, and, of course, rings – polished stones such as turquoise, amethyst, opal, lapis lazuli, and rose quartz were set into silver or gold with tiny open circles, beaded clusters, or florets often forming a frame around them.

Archibald Knox (1864–1953) was born, studied and taught on the Isle of Man until 1897, when he moved to London to lecture at three of its art colleges; by 1899 he was employed by Liberty & Co., designing an extensive array (over 400 pieces) of exquisite enameled or stone-set silver and gold jewelry (as well as silver and pewter objects in the "Cymric" and "Tudric" lines respectively) and eventually becoming their chief designer. His teaching and design specialty was Celtic ornament, and his distinctively smooth and usually symmetrically curving, interlaced patterns obviously derived from medieval Celtic stonework and illuminated manuscripts.

C.R. Ashbee (1863-1942) was an architect as well as a silver and jewelry designer. Probably his best-known creation was the Guild and School of Handicraft, which he founded in 1888 and which, although shortlived, was distinguished for its furniture and metalwork, and, above all, for its jewelry. Ashbee himself provided a great many of the designs, which included the peacock, delicate flowers, and a tiny sailing ship, the so-called "craft of the guild." Among the jewelry designers who were a part of the guild was Fred T. Partridge, whose exquisitely crafted works, especially his combs, echo French Art Nouveau jewels; his use of such materials as brass, shell, horn, and steel also reveal a kinship with his Gallic contemporaries. Partridge married May Hart, an enamelist of great skill whose use of the *plique-à-jour* technique, though not as elaborate as that of the European jewelers, was nevertheless expert and resulted in lovely pieces.

Another important English guild, the Artificers' Guild, was founded in 1901 by Nelson Dawson (1859-1942), in Chiswick in London, and was taken over two years later by Montague Fordham, erstwhile director of the Birmingham Guild of Handicraft. Along with his wife, Edith, Dawson created beautiful enameled jewelry, often decorated with floral and avian motifs. Dawson had learned the skill of enameling from Alexander Fisher, who was known for his plaques, sconces, and other large decorated pieces composed of layers of enamel on a foil ground.

Like many Arts and Crafts jewelers, another husband and wife team, Arthur and Georgina Gaskin, were connected with the city of Birmingham. Their inspirations and output were various – the former ranged from Italian Renaissance to Scandinavian folk art – and their pieces, whether a busily organic brooch with tiny enameled florets or a simple silver necklace pendant with green chrysoprase hearts, were all expertly crafted by hand.

Henry Wilson (1864-1934), like many other Arts and Crafts designers, initially studied and practiced architecture. He produced some exquisite pieces of jewelry at the turn of the century, inspired primarily by nature and the medieval and Renaissance past, and some extraordinary jewels, like earlier Italian masterworks, would feature stunning designs on both front and back.

Omar Ramsden (1873-1939) and Alwyn C. E. Carr (1872-1940) produced jewelry with religious overtones (this in addition to their more numerous metal ceremonial objects), and another significant teacher-designer-jewelry maker was Harold Stabler (1872-1945), much of whose cloisonné enamelwork, was made in collaboration with his wife, Phoebe, in his Hammersmith studio. Oliver Baker (1859-1939) and Jessie M. King (1875-1949) were two jewelry designers working for Liberty. Baker dis-

tinguished himself for his handsome silver buckle designs, usually hammered, with strong *entrelac* or curling motifs, and embellished with cabochons of semiprecious stones. King's Liberty jewels tend to betray their Glaswegian origins, especially her lovely enameled-silver belt buckles, whose florets nearly camouflage Charles Rennie Mackintosh-inspired birds amid their trelliswork.

Unlike objects in other fields, such as furniture, metalwork and pottery, fine American Arts and Crafts

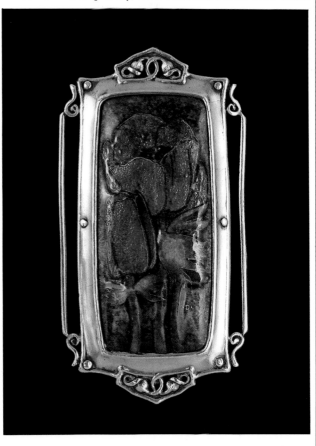

The enameled-silver belt buckle dates from the turn of the century and was made by Nelson and Edith Dawson. Floral motifs abounded on the Dawsons' hand-crafted pieces, whose surface and textures were purposefully matte and grainy, which gave them a quiet, gentle beauty. Nelson Dawson was the founder of the Artificers' Guild, established in Chiswick in 1901.

jewelry was a rarity; the Gallic Art Nouveau style seemed the greater influence on American jewelers, who in the main were companies rather than guilds or individual craftsmen. However, one firm, Marcus & Co., created some exquisite Arts and Crafts-style (or "crafts revival") jewelry in addition to Art Nouveau; and Florence Koehler, working in Chicago, fashioned pieces akin to those of her British contemporaries.

France, Belgium, and the United States

The Arts and Crafts Movement itself, as directly connected to Morris, was all but dead by the early 20th century. As its part in the decorative arts in Britain decreased, Art Nouveau was emerging, with all its waves

INTRODUCTION

and tendrils, *femmes fatales* and comely maidens, botanical verity and Symbolist allusions. There was the hyper-organic furniture and ironwork of Hector Guimard, the homage-to-nature glass and wood of Emile Gallé and Louis Majorelle, but most of all the exquisitely crafted, often dazzlingly pictorial goldsmith's work of René Lalique, Georges Fouquet, Lucien Gaillard, and other Parisian jewelers. Their acclaim was worldwide, their clients – such as actress Sarah Bernhardt and courtesan Liane de Pougy – world famous, and their influence permanent.

Unlike the subdued forms of Arts and Crafts jewelry, Art Nouveau jewelry could be dramatic, symbolic, ostentatious and, in the case of some of Lalique's massive chest ornaments, impractically overwhelming in size, weight, and impact. The types of jewelry worn ranged from diadems and combs, necklaces and pendants to shoe buckles, bracelets, stickpins, and rings; and the colors, materials and techniques were wildly diverse: there were precious, semiprecious and non-precious gems and metals, substances such as glass, horn, and tortoiseshell, and expert enameling of the translucent, opalescent, *champlevé,* cloisonné and *plique-à-jour* varieties.

Without doubt, the Frenchman René Lalique (1860–1945) was the master goldsmith of the Art Nouveau era. His one-off, exquisitely crafted rings, bracelets, dog-collars (decorative central plaques usually attached to ribbons or rows of pearls, and worn tightly across the neck), brooches, haircombs, necklaces, and tiaras were truly works of art, widely praised and exhibited in Europe and abroad, and,

inevitably, imitated in varying degrees of quality and imagination in France and elsewhere. Lalique's innovative joining of "lesser" materials with precious gems and metals and his rich use of natural, fantastic, literary, Neoclassical, oriental, Symbolist and even religious images combine to make his body of jewels a significant contribution to the art of the goldsmith, and to the decorative arts in general.

Although overshadowed by Lalique's highly imaginative, original, and widely varied designs, the goldsmith's work of several other Frenchmen in the Art Nouveau period ranks among the finest decorative work of that time. Noteworthy names include the Maison Vever (headed by the brothers, Paul and Henri, and employing such notable figures as the engraver Lucien Gautrait and the illustrator Eugène Grasset); Lucien Gaillard, who was much influenced by Japanese style and techniques; Eugène Feuillâtre, a skilled enamelist who had been apprenticed to Lalique; Georges Fouquet, whose firm commissioned Alphonse Mucha to design jewels for Sarah Bernhardt; Edward Colonna, who was born in Germany and who worked in France and the United States designing jewelry (and furniture) for Samuel Bing's Maison de l'Art Nouveau, as did Bing's son, Marcel; and Jules Desbois, whose chased-gold and silver brooches, buckles and buttons usually featured languorous female nudes or profiled faces in detailed bas-relief.

Numerous established jewelry firms, such as Boucheron, and newly founded retail companies like Julius Meier-Graefe's La Maison Moderne, produced handsome Art Nouveau pendants, brooches, combs and so on. The young Paul Follot and Maurice Dufrêne both designed heavily florid pieces for Meier-Graefe's Paris shop, and Théodore Lambert designed rather subdued floral and foliate pieces which were executed by Paul Templier and featured much openwork and filigree. In Belgium, Philippe Wolfers (1858–1929) designed outstanding work for the family firm, Wolfers Frères.

Across the Atlantic, several American jewelry-producing firms marketed wares highly reminiscent of French Art Nouveau. Foremost among these was the Gorham Corporation, founded in Providence, Rhode Island, in the early 19th century. Although Gorham employed many English designers in the 1800s, its trademarked "Martelé" jewelry, produced from around 1890, was often distinctly Gallic in feel. Unger Bros in Newark, New Jersey, also offered jewelry in the Art Nouveau style, most of it silver, sometimes lightly vermeiled. Other American firms producing Art Nouveau jewelry were Krementz (also in Newark) and Frank M. Whiting Company in North Attleboro, Massachusetts; while countless other costume jewelry firms in America – and Europe – produced pieces influenced by French designs (though often poorly executed by machine).

The maker of this Austrian pendant of c. 1910 is unknown, but it is an interesting Continental jewel featuring a Celtic interlace motif of silver, aquamarine, peridot, chrystoberyl, and a baroque pearl. The octagonal pendant may have been designed by a member of the Wiener Werkstätte.

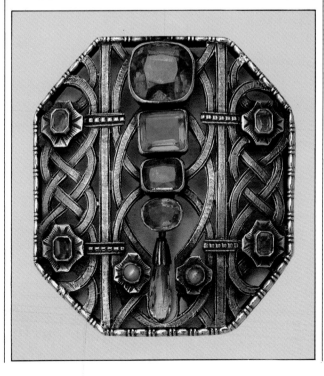

Tiffany & Co. in New York, founded in 1834, produced a small number of outstanding Art Nouveau jewelry pieces under the directorship of Louis Comfort Tiffany (1848–1933), better known for his stained-glass windows, Favrile glass, and leaded lamps. The "art jewelry" department was opened in 1902 under the supervision of Julia Munson; Louis Comfort himself designed necklaces, brooches, and other pieces, which often combined semiprecious and precious stones with glass or enamel-on-metal. Their style was more Revival or even Byzantine than that of typical Gallic Art Nouveau jewelry.

Moderne Jewelry in Germany and Austria

In Austria, where the *moderne* style took root rather early – in the last years of 19th century and the first decade or so of the 20th – some amazingly far-seeing pieces of jewelry were being designed by the likes of Josef Hoffmann, the architect, and his contemporaries. The Wiener Werkstätte dominated by circles, squares, and other geometric shapes; a square-framed Hoffmann brooch of silver, for instance, features a group of lapis lazuli cabochons in circular, square, rectangular, and triangular shapes, intermingling with tiny heart-shaped leaves. Jewels such as this were not mass-produced and occupy a significant place in early 20th-century jewelry design – neither Arts and Crafts nor Art Nouveau, but decidedly new and different. However, there were Austrian jewelers whose works distinctly echoed Gallic Art Nouveau, among them Franz Hauptmann and the firm of Rozet & Fischmeister.

Jugendstil ("Young Style") Germany proved a fertile ground for jewelry designers, with a huge output of pieces from, above all, Pforzheim, where the firm of Theodor Fahrner (1868–1928) mass-produced generally inexpensive jewels to the designs of Josef Maria Olbrich, Henry van de Velde, Moritz Gradl, Patriz Huber, and other designers allied to the Darmstadt artists' colony set up by the Grand Duke Ernst-Ludwig of Hesse, a supporter of the Arts and Crafts Movement. In other German cities – Munich, Dresden, Berlin – jewelry was being created in a variety of styles, from Lalique-like (by Robert Koch), to Wolfers-inspired (Theodor von Gosen), to distinctively Jugendstil, such as Berliner Hermann Hirzel's leafy gold forms designed by goldsmith Louis Werner.

On the whole, other European countries produced jewelry which either copied mainstream French pieces or adhered to indigenous provincial or unimaginatively traditional-European styles and forms. In Denmark, however, Mogens Ballin, Harald Slott-Müller, Eric Magnussen, and, above all, Georg Jensen distinguished themselves with their handsome designs. Jensen (1866–1935), a silversmith, potter, and sculptor, opened a jewelry atelier in Copenhagen in 1904, later producing large silver pieces such as coffeepots and trays in addition to his jewelry. His heavy silver brooches, combs, buckles and bracelets – some highlighted with cabochon amber or other semiprecious stones – featured stylized flowers, leaves, birds, and animals.

In Eastern Europe, too, the influence of French and Belgian designers could be seen, most visibly in the Art Nouveau-style goldsmith's work of the esteemed Russian firm of Peter Carl Fabergé. Curvilinear, organic forms adorned many a House of Fabergé bejeweled piece, but this was just one type of decoration they adopted – Revival and peasant styles being two others. In Budapest, while the designs of Oskar Huber reflected the more controlled curves of the German jewelers, their flattened *champlevé* enamelwork was akin to traditional, native techniques.

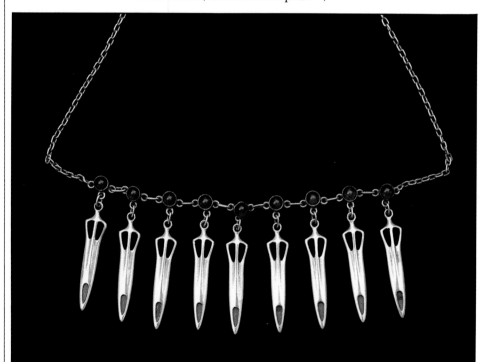

The Pforzheim firm of Theodor Fahrner produced a wide array of jewelry from the late 1800s well into the Art Deco era. Its designs came from both German and English sources, and, in fact, it made pieces marketed by the London wholesaler Murrle, Bennett & Co. (some with obvious British designs, giving rise to difficulties in their identification today). The lovely enameled-silver and amethyst necklace was made by Fahrner around 1905.

113

INFLUENCES

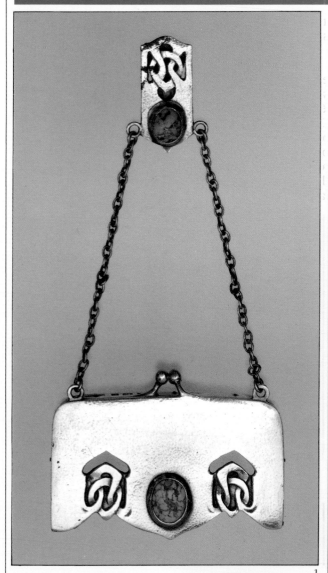

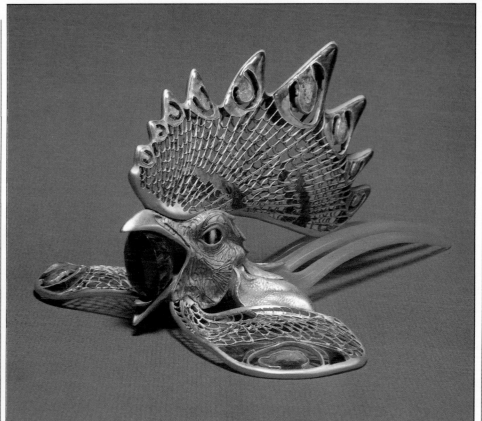

Many English Arts and Crafts designers were inspired by the motifs of the Middle Ages. The Celtic *entrelac* was often used by Archibald Knox, who designed the silver purse frame (*1*), set with turquoise matrix. Its interlace patterns are similar to those on the High Cross of Patrick and Columba (*2*) at Kells, in Ireland, 6th–7th century, and those on the decorative border of the silver, gold, copper, and amber- and glass-studded Ardagh Chalice (*3*), 8th century.

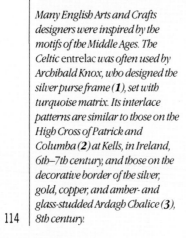

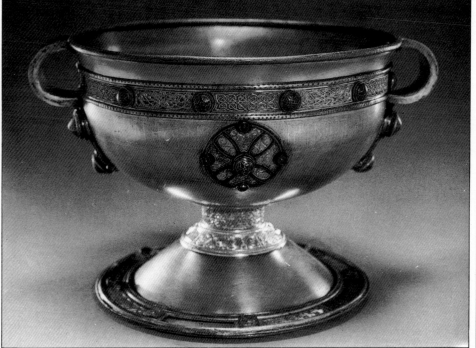

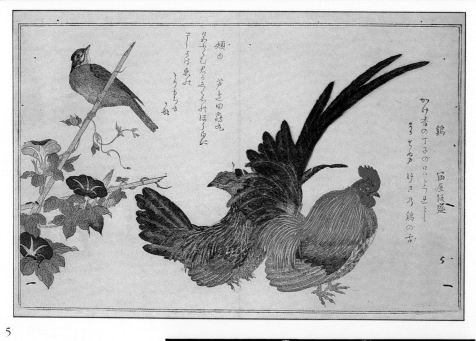

5

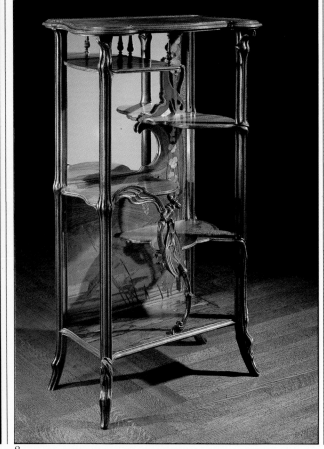

French Art Nouveau jewelers adopted imagery from sources as disparate as Symbolist poetry and Oriental prints. René Lalique created the stunning enameled-gold cock's head diadem (4); the magnificent bird's beak clutches an amethyst. It relates not only to the Utamaro illustration (5), from The Hundred Birds with Humorous Verses, *but also to the cloisonné enameled vase (6), from the Meiji period.*

6

Flora and fauna were represented in loving detail by many French Art Nouveau designers – on glass vases, on carved and inlaid furniture, and on goldsmith's work. Insects were especially favored by designers of the Ecole de Nancy: the étagère by Emile Gallé (8), with its monumental dragonfly support, is a superb, even somewhat monstrous, example of this entomological bent. On a smaller scale, René Lalique's delicate pendant (7) of gold, diamonds, and plique-à-jour enamel depicts a pair of facing grasshoppers – an exercise in both scientific and symmetrical precision.

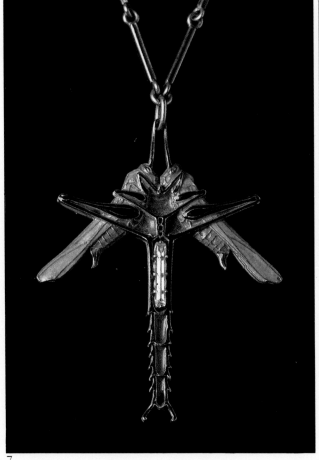

7

8

ANIMAL FORMS

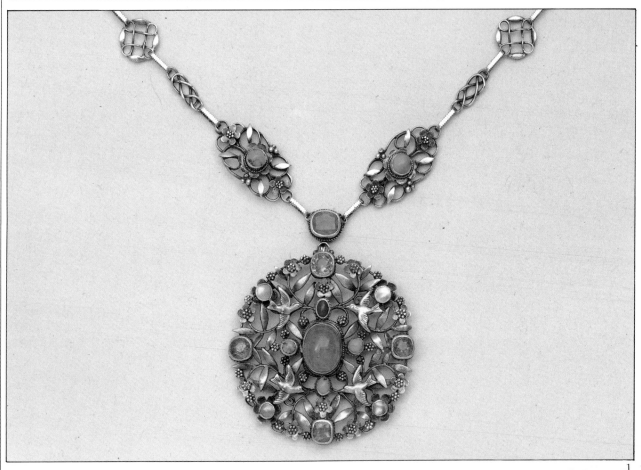

From the delicate and everyday to the monumental and grotesque, the range of creatures depicted on turn-of-the-century jewelry was vast. Even Arts and Crafts designers were not averse to decorating their pieces with the occasional bird or animal motif: the lovely creation (c. 1910) by Arthur and Georgina Gaskin (1) incorporates a quartet of tiny birds into its silver and silver-gilt pendant; tourmalines, mother-of-pearl, turquoise, and paste set off the metalwork. Another English jewel is the brooch by John Paul Cooper (2) comprising a golden stag amid a rock crystal, gold, and enamel roundel. The stunning ring tray (3) of c. 1900–1 was made by Eugène Feuillâtre, who for a time worked with René Lalique. Four silver serpents make up the frame of the piece, and its central section, of plique-à-jour enamel, features a colorful piscine creature in the Japoniste vein.

1

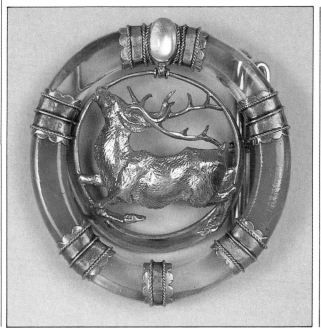

2

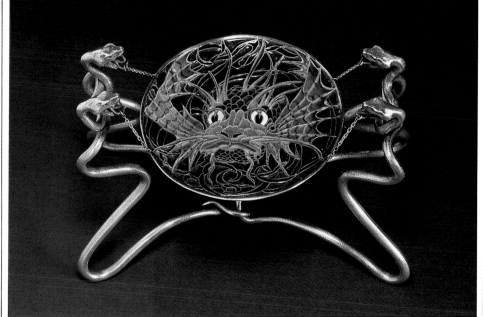

3

René Lalique's large and powerful jewels were often worn by women who were themselves larger than life – such as the actress Sarah Bernhardt and the celebrated dancer and courtesan Liane de Pougy, seen in a photograph of c. 1890–5 wearing a Lalique pendant and head ornament (**5**). The same oxidized-silver, enamel, and chrysoprase creation, converted into a brooch, is illustrated alone (**6**). The horrific winged dragon, in the Egyptian taste, was in fact inspired by the Divine Sarah herself, playing the part of Cleopatra.

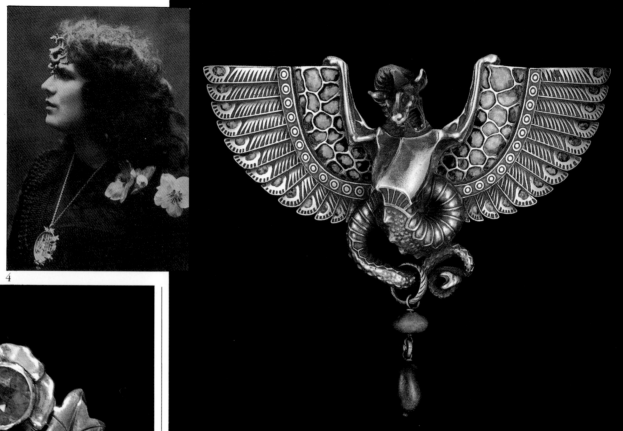

4

5

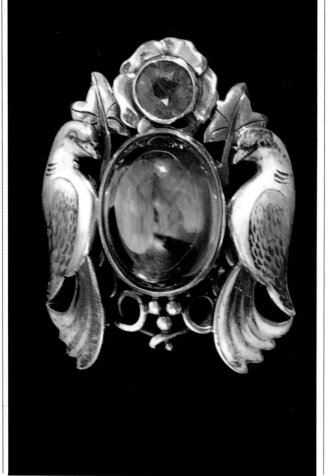

Birds were among the most popular creatures on British Arts and Crafts jewels, and the enameled-silver, amethyst, and peridot ring (**6**), probably by George Hunt, sports a strong avian design. Actually the ring most likely dates from the 1920s, but it is decidedly in the earlier Arts and Crafts mode. The silver and moonstone brooch (**7**) of c. 1910 by the Dane Georg Jensen has a central bird motif. As the moderne style came to dominate his silver, Jensen's animals became more stylized and simplified; this brooch, however, is in his earlier, somewhat heavier, style.

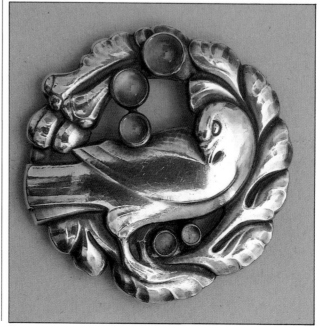

6   7

COMBS AND BUCKLES

THE JEWELRY OF LIBERTY & CO.

In 1875, Arthur Lasenby Liberty (1843–1917) opened a small retail shop on London's Regent Street and called it East India House; he specialized in selling Oriental fabrics and goods, including silks from India and porcelain and screens from Japan. By 1885, the shop had expanded considerably and become extremely popular. Besides importing exotic goods, Liberty was now commissioning English designers to create fabrics, fashions, furniture, pottery, and other wares for his shop. At the turn of the century, Liberty & Co. imported, commissioned, and sold a huge variety of native, other European, and Oriental goods; silver and pewter objects were added to the inventory in the 1890s (sold under the tradenames "Cymric" and "Tudric," respectively), and included a large number of jewelry pieces. Although Liberty insisted on maintaining a policy of anonymity for his designers, his employees – among them

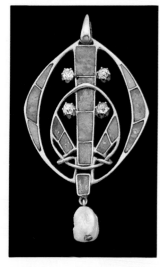

Gold, opal, and pearl pendant by Archibald Knox for Liberty & Co.

Archibald Knox, Jessie M. King, Bernard Cuzner, Oliver Baker, Arthur and Georgina Gaskin, and Rex Silver – were some of the most prominent names in Arts and Crafts design of the time. The buckles, waist clasps, brooches, pendants, bracelets, rings, necklaces, and other Liberty pieces – of smooth or hammered silver and sometimes gold, highlighted with rich enameling, moonstones, turquoise, opals, mother-of-pearl, etc. – were distinguished for their innovative designs and color combinations. The Celtic interlace pattern (attributable to Knox) was perhaps Liberty's best-known motif, but stylized flowers, heart-shaped leaves, and loose, sometimes asymmetrical tendrils akin to those of Gallic goldsmiths' work were also a part of the vast Liberty repertoire. Besides employing domestic jewelry designers and manufacturers, Liberty also bought designs from companies in Pforzheim, Germany, a major jewelry-making center. Technically, Liberty's factory-made commercial jewels (some with hand-finishing) cannot be deemed Arts and Crafts, as can the hand-crafted creations of the various English artisan guilds, yet many of their designs especially Knox's interlaced pieces, do relate to the spirit of the Arts and Crafts Movement.

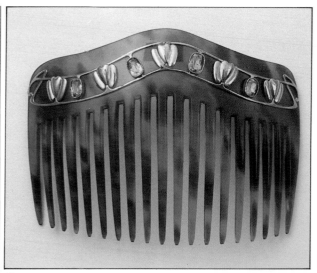

Haircombs were a popular accessory at the turn of the century. Some, like the Murrle, Bennett & Co. design (2), were simply shaped, displaying period elements in their added design: here heart-shaped gold leaves alternate with peridots on a tortoiseshell ground.

1

A long-toothed horn, gold, enamel, and opal comb (1) by the Parisian Georges Fouquet, ambitiously carved as evidenced by the openwork motif of stylized lotus blossoms.

2

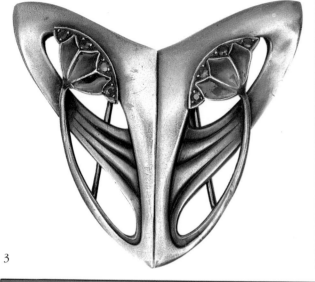

3

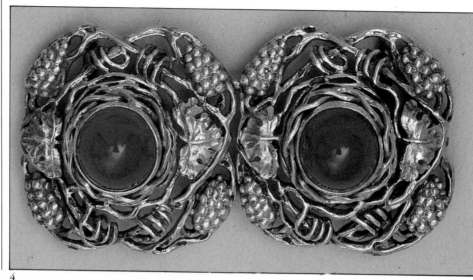

4

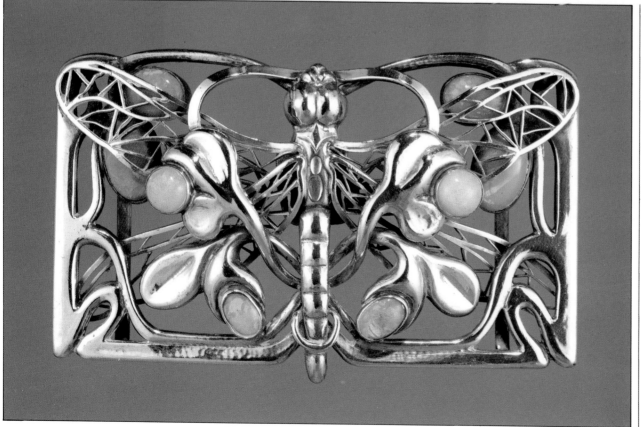

5

Some of the loveliest Arts and Crafts and Art Nouveau jewels were belt buckles, or clasps for joining together the sides of the heavy cloaks that were so often worn at the turn of the century. The handsome silver plique-à-jour enamel and paste buckle (**3**), c. 1905, is probably German or Austrian. Its strong, curved design is typically Jugendstil, but its stylized lotus blossoms add a colorful, delicate touch. Joseph Hodel, who was associated with the Bromsgrove Guild of Applied Art in England, designed the silver and chrysoprase buckle (**4**), with its dense but organized massing of grapes, leaves, and encircling tendrils. The chef d'oeuvre (**5**) by Danish silversmith Georg Jensen dates from c. 1904. Jensen has borrowed a popular motif from his French contemporaries, the dragonfly, and stylized it in his own idiomatic way, using silver, opals, and native techniques to produce an arresting, outstanding piece.

MEDIEVAL INFLUENCES

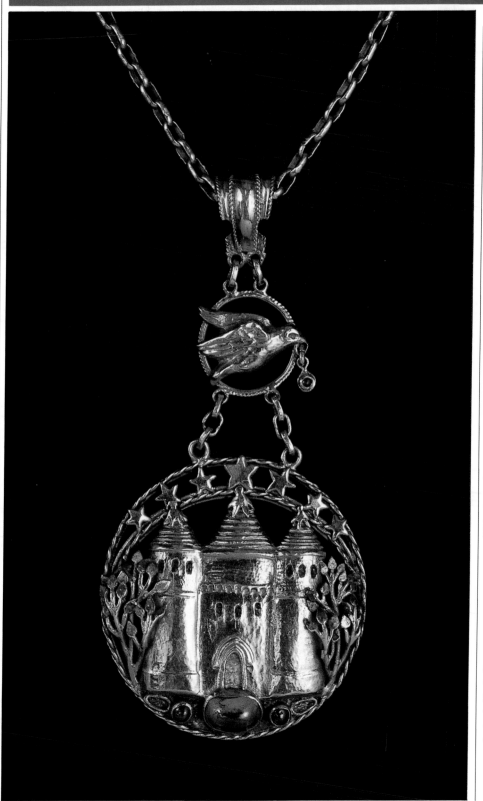

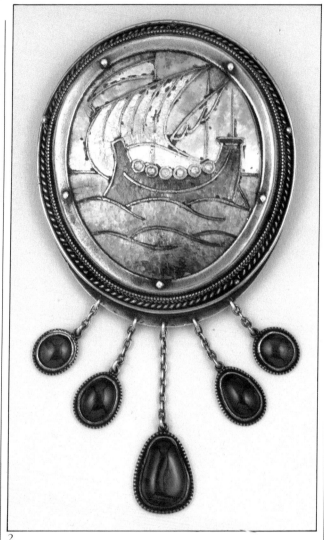

2

Many Arts and Crafts jewelers
looked to the Middle Ages (and
sometimes the Renaissance) for
inspiration regarding materials,
techniques, and subjects. Two
lovely pictorial pieces are the silver,
enamel, and garnet brooch (**2**),
possibly by the Guild of Handicraft,
and the gold, enamel, and stone
pendant (**1**), by John Paul Cooper.
Both these English designs have
medieval subjects: a Viking sailing
ship and a turreted castle.

1

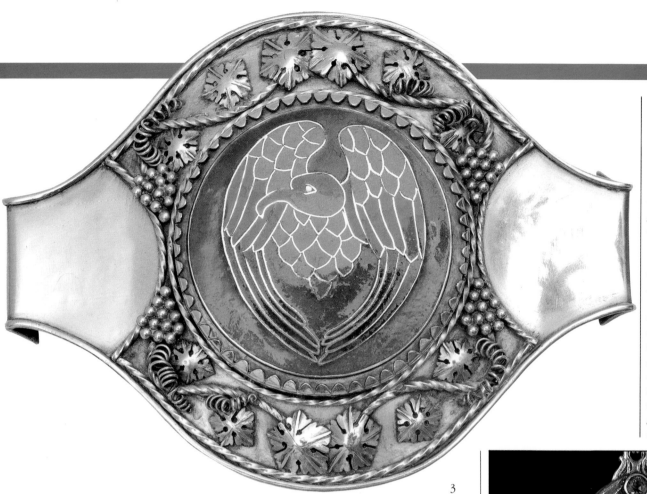

3

The substantial belt buckle (3) of silver and cloisonné enamel resembles a medieval shield, complete with stylized aquiline motif. Its typical Arts and Crafts border of leaves, grape clusters, and tendrils, however, firmly places it in this mode (it is attributed to Harold Stabler, c. 1910). Yet another medievalizing design is the silver and enamel pendant (5) by the Englishman Omar Ramsden, c. 1900; its form is like that of a religious triptych, and indeed its central section features a saint bearing shield and sword. Somewhat surprising is René Lalique's wonderful usage of a medieval subject, a couple wearing period headdresses, in a gold, ivory, sapphire, enamel, and diamond pendant, c. 1900–2 (4).

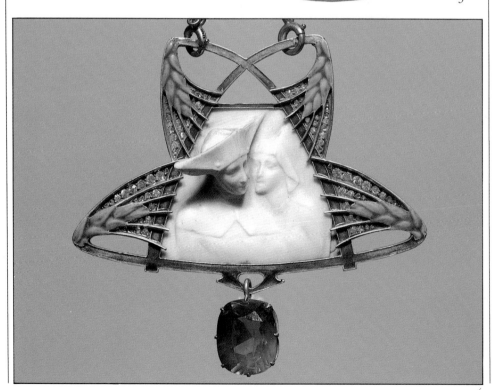

4

5

FIGURATIVE PIECES

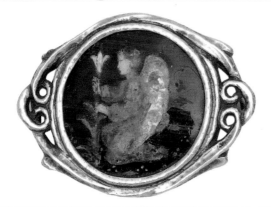

1

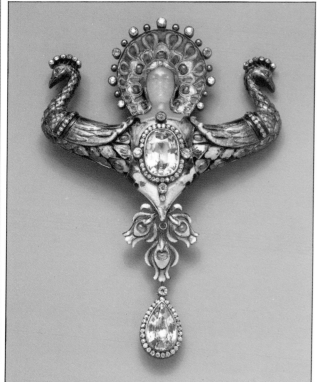

2

Art Nouveau is noted for its depictions of women – usually languorous, long-dressed beauties, but sometimes more sublime, ethereal types, or even femmes fatales. An elaborate bodice adornment (3) features the quintessential Art Nouveau woman; indeed, the gold, enamel, emerald, and baroque pearl piece, its figure painted on mother-of-pearl, is a combined effort by the premier illustrator of the time, Czech-born Alphonse Mucha, and goldsmith Georges Fouquet. A more enigmatic female is flanked by a pair of peacocks in a yellow sapphire, diamond, jade, and enamel pendant (2). A silver and enamel brooch depicting an androgynous angel (1), by the Englishwoman Ernestine Mills, is dated 1918, but is very much in the early Arts and Crafts manner.

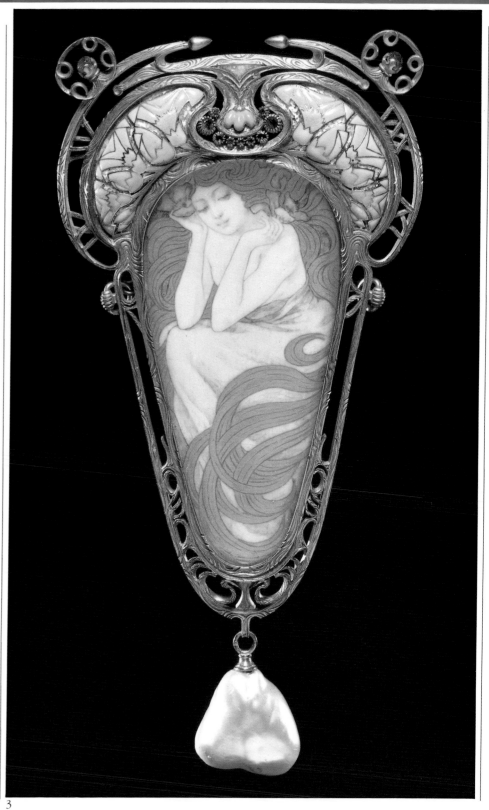

3

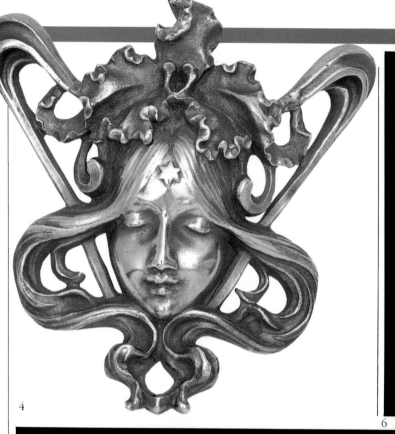

4

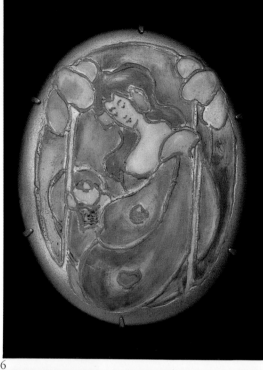

6

The long-haired, lovely woman in a variety of fin-de-siècle guises appears in the three jewels on this page. The silver brooch (**4**) depicts an orchid-bedecked head, the eyes closed in reverie, a six-pointed star marking the brow. The unusual painted-ceramic brooch (**6**) c.1910, is by the Englishman Thomas A. Cook, who was also known for his figural fan designs; the woman on this pin is simply painted and vaguely Oriental in appearance. A stunning angelic head is in the center of a brooch of 1904 by Parisian Georges Fouquet (**5**). Second only to Lalique for his goldsmith's work, Fouquet has fashioned here a mystery-laden masterpiece, replete with halo, wings, and lotus blossoms, out of gold, enamel, opal, glass, diamonds, and pearls.

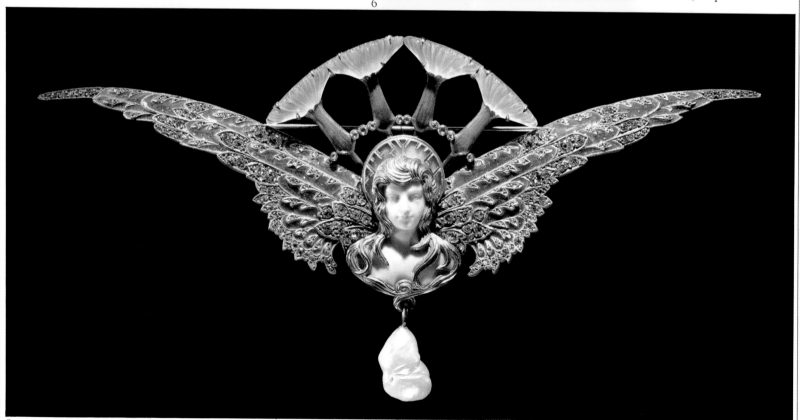

5

BOTANICAL FORMS

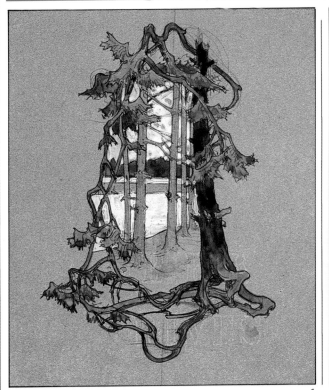

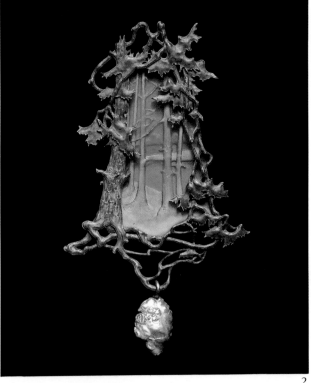

From simple, stylized blossoms to detailed, realistic landscapes, nature in all her forms, real and imaginary, was represented on both Art Nouveau and Arts and Crafts jewelry. René Lalique transformed gold, enamel, and glass into a stunning winter-woodland pendant (c. 1899–1900) (**2**), an icy baroque pearl suspended from the lower branches of its tree frame. Landscape with Trees on the Bank of a Lake (**1**) by René Lalique; pencil, pen and ink and gouache on paper is its preliminary design. The Scotswoman Jessie M. King created this charming silver and enamel pendant (**3**) for Liberty & Co., c. 1902.

1

2

The turquoise matrix, gold, and enamel brooch (**4**) was designed by C.R. Ashbee for the Guild of Handicraft, c. 1899. In fact, it is in the shape of a butterfly, but it can be interpreted as a somewhat floriform design also.

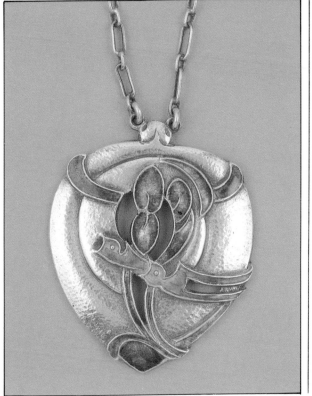

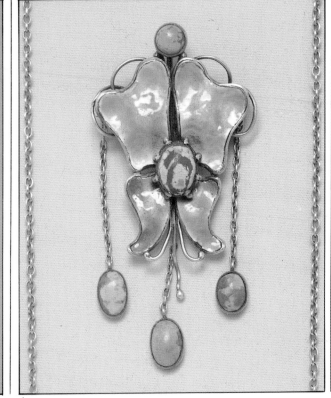

3

4

The long career of Scottish-born Sybil Dunlop began in the early 20th century and lasted until the late 1930s. Out of her studio-shop on Kensington Church Street, in London, came a plethora of handsome jewels, all hand-fashioned in the Arts and Crafts vein, but the later pieces tinged with Dunlop's unique brand of modernism. This brooch (**5**), probably of the 1920s, features rich masses of silver, silver-gilt, stones, and paste amid the leafy, beaded clusters and coiled tendrils common in early Arts and Crafts goldsmith's work.

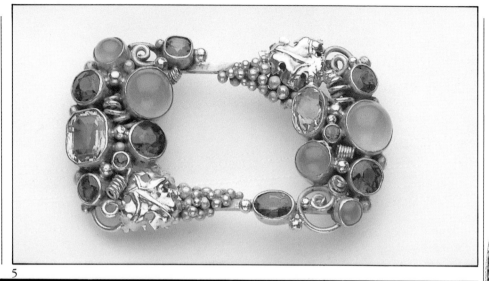

5

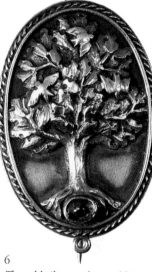

6

The gold, silver, and emerald Tree of Life brooch (**6**), c. 1905–10, is probably by John Paul Cooper or Edward Spencer, English goldsmiths who worked in a medievalizing manner. The fecund tree is richly detailed, down to the trio of birds amid its leaves. Conversely, the silver, malachite, agate, and pearl brooch by Viennese Carl Otto Czeschka (**7**) is rich in simple, spare stylization. The juxtaposition of the large blossom and the huge stones is jarring, but fin-de-siècle Viennese design did indeed anticipate Art Deco with its bold modernism.

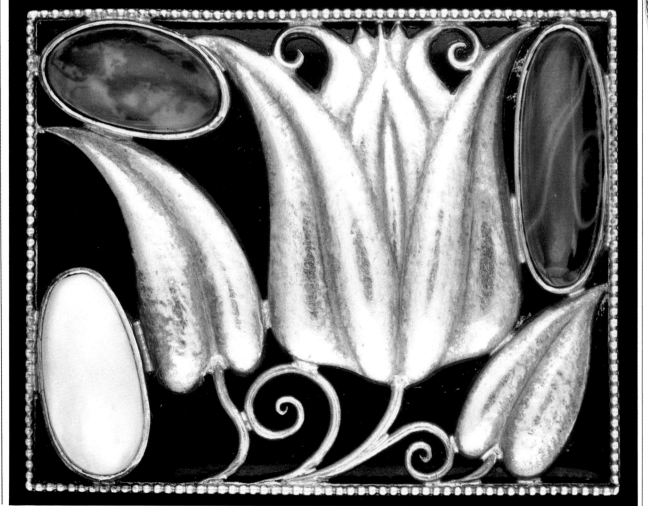

7

TECHNIQUES

The methods of jewelry making employed by the great Art Nouveau goldsmiths were highly sophisticated; their mixture of precious and semiprecious stones and metals was innovative as well, although it soon became commonplace. The maker of the buckle (*1*) was probably French; its workmanship is more primitive than that of the best Gallic jewelry; but the buckle's combination of silver-gilt, seed and baroque pearls, and plique-à-jour enamel is typically French (this technique essentially resembles stained glass: its different sections are separated by wires, and it has no background).

A similar effect to that of plique-à-jour enamel is seen on the lovely gold and opal necklace (*3*) designed by Archibald Knox for Liberty & Co. The opal segments, arranged in a mosaic-like pattern, and the openwork sections in between, make for a novel and sophisticated design, quite different from Knox's applied-enamel pieces.

The totally hand-fashioned brooch (*2*) from the Guild of Handicraft was designed by C.R. Ashbee, its founder, c. 1902–3. Of gold, enamel, and turquoise, it features a sailing ship enhanced with lovely applied decoration, from twisted-gold ropes to a fluttering standard.

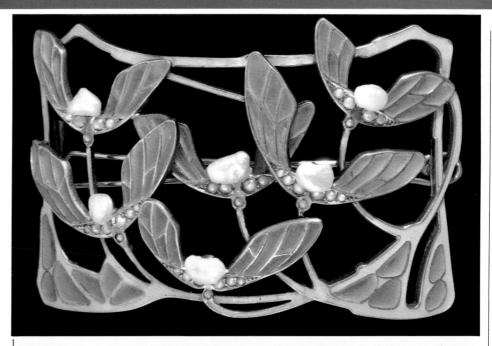

1

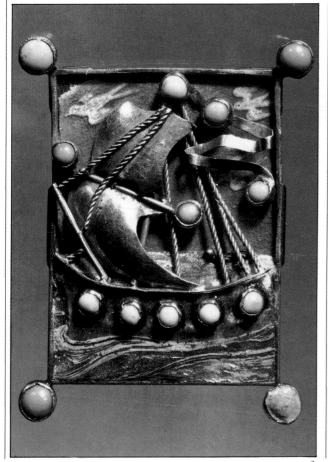

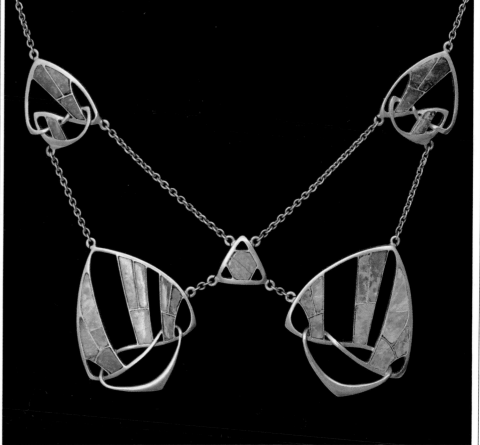

2 3

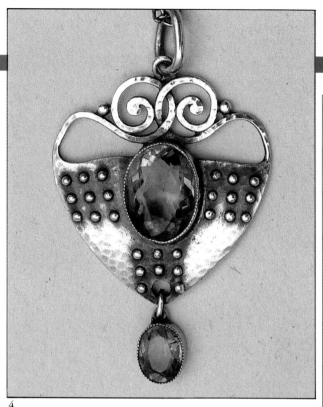

The silver and amethyst pendant (**4**) was marketed by the London wholesaler Murrle, Bennett & Co., but made in Pforzheim, a major jewelry-manufacturing center in Germany. Its intertwined scrolls, cruciform shape, applied studs, and hammered surface all relate to medieval sources. Though it is factory made, its hammering would have been done by hand.

Jessie M. King designed this silver and enamel belt buckle (**5**) for Liberty & Co. in 1906. Its two abstract birds are adapted from a design by the Glasgow architect-designer Charles Rennie Mackintosh, but the six stylized blossoms are typical of the many-talented King.

4

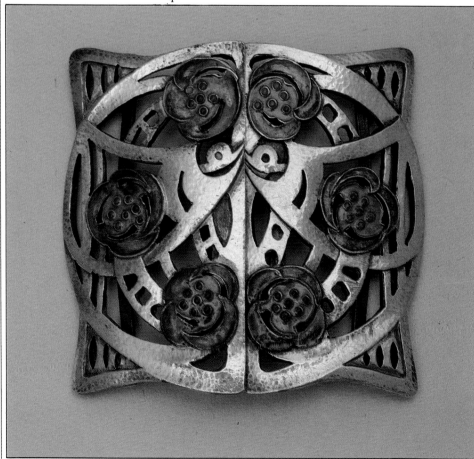

5

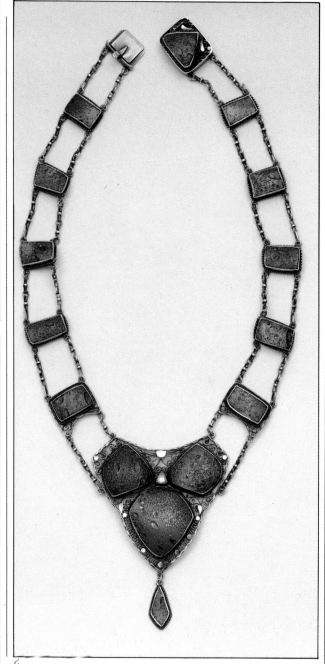

6

The highly unusual necklace (**6**) is of silver set with diamonds and plaques of the type of glass known as "Lava" which was made by Louis Comfort Tiffany. The necklace may have been fashioned by Tiffany, who opened an "art jewellery" department in the family firm, Tiffany & Co., in 1902. Though short-lived (it closed in 1916), it produced some lovely "art jewels" in the Crafts Revival, Byzantine style.

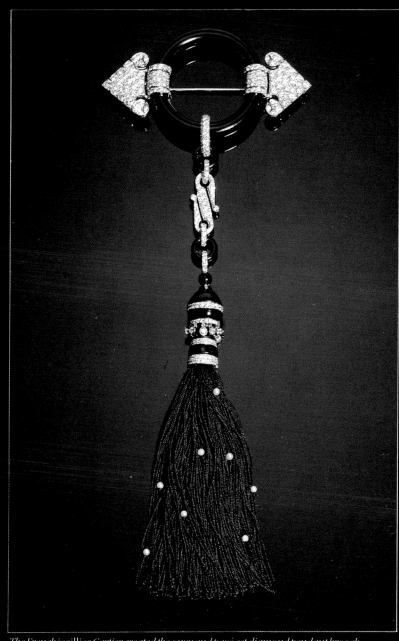

The French joaillier Cartier created the onyx and pavé-set diamond pendant brooch, with its pearl-scattered, detachable tassel. A quintessentially moderne jewel, it contains strong Art Deco features: a sense of geometry, a black-and-white color scheme, a combination of precious and non-precious substances, even a silk-fringe fillip (so much a part of that era's fashion, in both couture and interior design).

CHAPTER SEVEN

ART DECO

1920-1939

Following the Bauhaus

·

Innovative materials

·

France at its zenith

PATRICIA BAYER

INTRODUCTION

An intricately fashioned essay in geometry, this 1930s gilded-metal necklace has a strong Machine Age feel. Its stepped sections also relate to stepped Aztec pyramids, an architectural source for some Art Deco jewelry designers. The maker of the necklace is unknown, but the piece is French.

The jewelers of the Art Deco period, which lasted roughly from 1920 to 1939, produced some of the most dazzling pieces ever seen – daring, flamboyant, pristine, and even playful. This was the era of the flapper, the Jazz and Machine ages, the between-the-wars (but sandwiching-the-Depression) decades of carefreeness and, concurrently, conservatism, and the artistic output of the period reflected this variety. Unlike the Art Nouveau and Arts and Crafts periods, when noted designers held prime positions and exerted strong influences on other individuals and firms, the Art Deco years were strong on design itself, with many quintessential pieces anonymously designed, unsigned (except for perhaps a retailer's mark), and indeed even of uncertain national origin. So wide-ranging and pervasive a style was Art Deco that similar pieces – necklaces of, say, Bakelite and chrome – were being manufactured in places as disparate as New Jersey and Czechoslovakia.

Materials used by Art Deco jewelry makers ranged from the traditional and precious – diamonds (mostly baguette-cut), rubies, gold, pearls – to the unorthodox and innovative – plastic, chrome, steel. Sturdy, flexible platinum, which was first widely used in the late 19th century, was a relatively new luxury metal which worked well as a setting for emeralds, sapphires, and other precious gems, but also complemented such popular semiprecious opaque stones as coral, jade, onyx, and lapis lazuli. Costume jewelry, especially with the imprimaturs of the trendsetting couturières Coco Chanel and Elsa Schiaparelli, became ever more popular, outrageous, and acceptable – from garish paste chokers and earrings to comical plastic-fish bangles and (from Schiaparelli) a colored-metal Zodiac-sign necklace.

In the 1920s and 30s, a wide range of jewelry was worn: dangling rhinestone earrings, which showed off the short bobbed haircuts of the Roaring Twenties; bracelets and bangles, the latter often worn en masse on bare upper arms; ultra-long beaded *sautoirs,* which complemented the dropped waistlines of the 1920s; prominent pendants to adorn newly revealed *décolletés* and backs; ubiquitous and multipurpose clips – geometric, floral, figural, and usually in pairs – which the 1930s woman attached to her shoes, hat, collar, belt, and so on.

The myriad influences contributing to Art Deco jewelry design came from Pharaonic Egypt, the Orient, tribal Africa, Cubism, and Futurism; from machines and graphic design; even from buildings, such as stepped Mayan temples and their latter-day descendants, the big-city skyscrapers. Images of animals of speed and grace –the greyhound, the gazelle, and the deer – as well as of new-fangled automobiles and airplanes were found on both precious and mass-produced jewels. Human subjects were not as common as on Art Nouveau goldsmith's work, but some noted designers depicted them in their works, and,

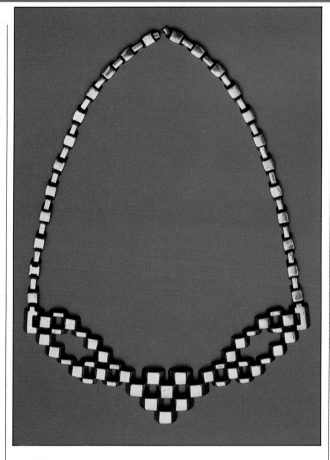

more often, they appeared on inexpensive, anonymous baubles. René Lalique, who created glass jewelry in the 1920s and 30s (having first achieved fame as the premier Art Nouveau goldsmith), molded some of his pendants with romantic women; stylized African heads formed brooches by Chanel and others; Emile Davide depicted handsome Neo-classical figures, and stylish 1920s women were cut from cheap white metals, sometimes attached by tiny chains to modish canines.

Most of all, however, jewelry of the 1920s and 30s was in thrall to geometry – to circles, arcs, squares, rectangles, triangles, and so on, singly and in combination, sometimes pure and unadorned, sometimes slightly embellished to become stylized flowers or leaves or sunbursts, some of pure metal, others of set cabochon stones. Scrolls, ribbons and more elaborate but still relatively uncomplicated forms appear as well, especially in the 1930s. (In the 1940s they would get heavier and chunkier.)

The Art Jewelers of Paris

Paris, of course, was both the source and the trendsetter of Art Deco, which is itself named after the 1925 Exposition des Arts Décoratifs et Industriels Modernes held in Paris. In fact, as early as the 1910s and up to the 1930s it was the fount of innovative fashion; it follows that Paris should have led the way in *moderne* jewelry.

The Swiss-born designer Jean Dunand (1877–1942), whose hammered-metal and lacquered vases and lacquered furniture and screens were greatly indebted to Asian and other non-Western styles, also designed a small but stunning body of jewelry. Largely of silver lacquered with red and black, Dunand's dangling earrings and earclips, brooches, and bracelets, assumed geometric shapes containing equally strong motifs – interwoven or superimposed lines, zigzags, openwork squares, and triangles, and so on. Their kinship with the painting of the time is immediately evident, and indeed Dunand often collaborated with the Cubist painter and sculptor Jean Lambert-Rucki on his larger projects.

Gérard Sandoz (b. 1902) came from a family of jewelers and began to design starkly geometric pieces for the Sandoz firm while still a teenager. His goldsmith's *oeuvre* dates from a period of just under a decade, yet his output is nonetheless significant within the realm of Art Deco jewelry. The clean lines and delicate craftsmanship of Sandoz's undeniably Machine Age pieces contributed to their significant place in the Art Deco repertoire.

Another gifted goldsmith was Jean Desprès (1889–1980), whose industrial-design training in the First World War is reflected in his strong pieces. His Machine Age aesthetic may be interpreted as unwieldy and masculine, but it was well suited to the Jazz Age, to the increasingly strong image of the liberated, at times androgynous, woman. In the late 1920s, Desprès started working with the Surrealist artist Etienne Cournault, whose engraved and painted motifs – one brooch featured a stylized lizard – on mirror-glass added a new design element to Desprès's earlier, more rigid pieces. Indeed, Desprès's modernist, industrial-derived pieces (and their contemporary and latter-day imitations) are some of the most desirable for collectors (and wearers) of vintage jewelry today.

Raymond Templier (1891–1968), like Sandoz, came from a family of Parisian jewelers, Maison Templier having been started by his grandfather in the mid–19th century. Templier's designs, like Desprès's, were boldly geometric, but sported more precious stones, for instance brooches with scatterings of diamonds against stark platinum fields. Templier was especially fond of precious white metals – platinum and silver – and paired them with onyx and other dark stones in stunning pieces (these were regarded as black and white color combinations, and were wildly popular in the Art Deco period). His designs for the actress Brigitte Helm's jewels in the film *L'Argent*, were marvelously theatrical, especially the blatantly architectonic ear pendants which could be miniature Empire State Buildings or John Storrs sculptures. Templier collaborated

with the designer Michel Percheron and at least once with the Cubist sculptor–painter Gustave Miklos, whose delicate plaster model of an elongated head he translated into a brooch of white and yellow gold.

Paul-Emile Brandt was a Swiss-born jeweler who began working in the Art Nouveau period but evolved into a highly admired Art Deco designer. His cocktail watches, for instance, are richly bejeweled yet strictly geometric. Finally, the Boivin atelier is also worth mentioning here. Opened in 1892 by René Boivin (who later married couturier Paul Poiret's sister, Jeanne), the firm produced handsome *mod-*

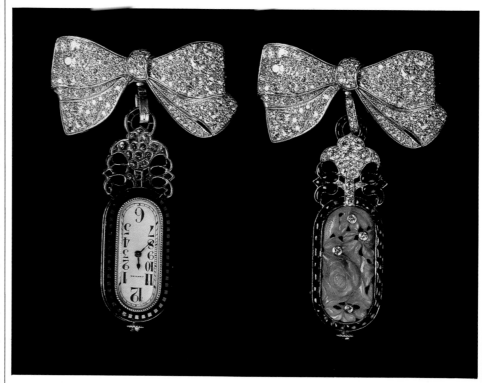

erne designs in the Art Deco period, under the direction of Madame Boivin and her two daughters (René had died in 1917).

The output of these "art jewelers" was small but significant in term of Art Deco design. Much more prolific, and in turn influential, were the mostly long established jewelry firms producing deluxe pieces – Cartier, Boucheron, Janesich, Chaumet, Mellerio, Fouquet, Vever and Van Cleef & Arpels.

Georges and Jean Fouquet were father and son, and both created outstanding Art Deco jewels. Georges (1862–1957), who had also produced Art Nouveau goldsmith's work for La Maison Fouquet (founded by his father, Alphonse), tended toward busy designs, whereas Jean Fouquet (b. 1899), leaned to more geometric forms *à la* Templier's and Sandoz's "art jewels." The Fouquet firm also

Wearable timepieces of all sorts – wristwatches, pendant watches, lapel-brooch watches – were worn by men and women of fashion and means in the Art Deco era. The firm of Louis Cartier, who is credited with the invention of the wristwatch in 1904, fashioned the pendant watch of diamonds, jade, onyx, and sapphires; it hangs from a diamond-encrusted bow (both front and back are shown).

commissioned jewelry from Eric Bagge, the noted architect and interior designer; painter André Leveillé; and the premier poster artist–illustrator of the day, A. M. Cassandre.

The Cartier firm, founded in 1847, reached dizzying heights of Art Deco splendor under the direction of Louis Cartier (1875–1942), whose fascination with exotic motifs led to the creation of diamond, ruby, and platinum earrings from which hung jade roundels carved with elephants, and a gold and enamel bangle with two carved-coral chimera heads facing each other in the center. In the 1930s, figural clips and brooches, featuring ornate blackamoor heads, even American Indian squaws and chiefs, were marketed by Cartier and spawned a whole wave of cheap imitations, especially in plastics and base metals. A great deal of carved jade and coral was used on Cartier's rings, brooches, jabot pins, bracelets, and necklaces, and motifs such as heavily bejeweled baskets or swags of flowers, berries, and leaves (popularly known as "fruit salads" or "tutti frutti") were composed of rich, colorful masses of carved emeralds, rubies, and sapphires amid variously cut and set diamonds. Geometric, or quasi-geometric, arrangements of diamonds, with gemstone highlights, also abounded. Of course, such motifs worked their way into the ever-growing repertoire of costume jewelry, too, with French, American, Czechoslovakian, and other factories flooding the market with paste resembling diamonds, rubies, emeralds, even onyx and jade.

The glass jewelry of René Lalique and Gabriel Argy-Rousseau deserves special mention. By the 1920s, the master goldsmith Lalique had become the premier glassmaker of France, and though his main output consisted of vases, tableware and figures, he also created some lovely glass jewelry: pendants, some inspired by openwork Japanese swordguards, or *tsubas,* and molded with stylized leaf or animal designs, others with insects and lovely female figures, all hanging from silk cords terminating in rich tassels; all-glass rings, molded with tiny flowers; expandable bracelets of wide rectangular sections decorated with stylized organic designs; necklaces made up partly or wholly of hemispherical, zigzag, floral, foliate, or round beads; and brooches on metal backs (often with colored foil in between) depicting subjects as varied as moths, a satyr, serpents, and a grazing stag. *Pâte-de-verre* master Argy-Rousseau also produced jewelry: one diamond-shaped pendant shows a white elephant in a leafy surround; a round medallion features a curtsying ballerina amid a floral border; and another pendant, this one oval, has three scarab beetles, one of many Egyptian motifs made popular in the 1920s following the discovery of Tutankhamun's tomb.

Among the other well-known deluxe jewelers, Mauboussin was noted for his highly colorful pieces, often set in black enamel; Boucheron continued to make great use of the diamonds which made them famous in the late

19th century, only now they were literally combined with lapis lazuli, jade, coral, onyx, and other semiprecious stones; and the jewels of Lacloche Frères, Chaumet, Linzeler & Marshak, Dusausoy, and so many other firms sparkled their way into the jewel boxes and onto the necks, arms, and clothes of the fashionable rich.

Motifs: from the sublime to the ridiculous

As for precious jewelry in the Art Deco style in other European countries, the little there was was largely derivative, like the Italian G. Ravasco's diamond-studded geometric creations or Theodor Fahrner's later jewels (Fahrner's factory in Pforzheim, Germany, mass-produced Arts and Crafts-style pieces earlier in the century). Some London jewelers, like Asprey and Mappin & Webb, produced Art Deco-style confections, but these are largely unsigned, so the designers are unknown. Some British designers however, like Sybil Dunlop, Harold Stabler and H.G. Murphy, known primarily for their Arts

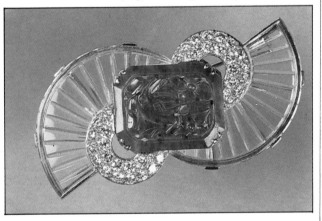

and Crafts-style pieces, produced decidedly *moderne* (though not geometric) jewels.

Georg Jensen's firm in Copenhagen continued to produce silver jewelry in the Art Deco era (and some gold as well), adding sharp geometric forms to its repertoire of stylized motifs. Animal subjects, especially the ever-popular deer, as well as flowers and leaves, adorned brooches, bracelets and buckles, and these in turn were imitated by a host of European and American jewelers.

The indigenous Mexican silver industry was highlighted in the Art Deco era via the talents of an American architect–designer–teacher, William Spratling, who settled in Taxco in 1929. He opened a shop dealing in traditional crafts and also started a school where he trained natives to work with silver and other local substances. Spratling produced some stunning brooches, bracelets, and earrings, mostly in silver set with amethysts, but some of gold, all of which had a clean, crisp quality which was highly sympathetic to the native materials used. A whole community of jewelers

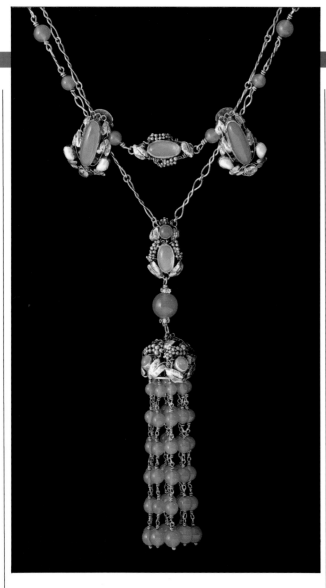

jewelry – diamond wedding rings in handsome geometric settings of platinum, bar pins and pendants with stepped designs, watches with colored-paste embellishments. Of course, there were American jewelers akin to Cartier (which had a New York branch, as did Van Cleef & Arpels and others). Some of them even had designs made up in Paris for them. In the main, precious American Art Deco *bijoux* tended to be more colorful than their Gallic counterparts.

Geometric rings, clips, brooches, bracelets, lapel watches, and necklaces abounded, of precious metals and jewels as well as of base metals or new alloys, paste, marcasite, plastic, and stones such as dark red carnelian and apple-green chrysoprase –both chalcedonies, and cheaper to use than coral and jade, which they resembled.

Costume jewelry of the 1920s and 30s – lovely, imaginative, fun, or all three – has surely come into its own in the recent past. In its own time, the fact that Coco Chanel and Elsa Schiaparelli, among other notables, were designing and sporting "fabulous fakes" made them desirable to a wide public. Today, the rage for antique or recent-vintage jewelry has made these 60 to 70-year-old pieces even more popular (though less and less affordable).

The motifs of Art Deco costume jewels range from the sublime to the ridiculous: from stunning geometric configurations of paste to silly plastic cherries dangling from a wooden bar. The serious pieces borrowed their subjects from deluxe jewelry of the time; the jokey style came about more or less on its own. Animals and people inhabit the world of 1920s and 30s costume jewelry, from gentle silver fawns and playful plastic Scottie dogs to paste, turquoise, and marcasite Chinamen and elegant, gilt-metal, cloche-hatted vamps. Flowers in every possible color, combination, and variety sprouted on gilt-metal or silver brooches and pendants, their paste petals glittering shamelessly.

In the late 1930s, sophisticated yet freeform designs began to appear (in both fine and costume jewelry, but especially the latter), with ribbons, bows, loops, and scrolls the predominant motifs. The Napier and Coro companies in the United States were at the forefront of the manufacture of these "cocktail jewels," which were highly kinetic and full of energy, unlike the more serene, decorative pieces of a decade or so earlier.

The Scottish-born Londoner Sybil Dunlop, many of whose handcrafted jewels reflect her Arts and Crafts training, created most of her pieces in the Art Deco era. The long 1930s necklace with tassel pendant and two matching clips, is indeed rife with Arts and Crafts materials and motifs – silver, chrysoprase, moonstone, leafy clusters, coiling wires – but its extreme length, moderne style, and beaded tassel are very much of the Jazz Age.

sprang up in Taxco around Spratling and his wife.

Many American jewelers and retailers made and marketed precious objects in the high-style French vein. These included Oriental-inspired pieces, like a bracelet from Marsh and Co. (a San Francisco jeweler), its carved-coral plaques alternating with iron sections enclosing Chinese characters; architectonic confections, like a pair of gold Tiffany clips comprising stepped sections of tiny squares, and Egyptian Revival baubles, such as Marcus & co.'s opal brooch with an elaborate gold setting featuring a Pharaoh and his queen, a scarab beetle, and lotus flowers.

Though French designs were often slightly toned down for wealthy, conservative clients, several significant jewelry manufacturers such as New York's Oscar Heyman & Brothers, the Bonner Manufacturing Company, and Walter P. McTeigue, Inc., provided Saks Fifth Avenue and other fine department stores with their creations. Even the mail-order Sears, Roebuck catalog featured *moderne*

INFLUENCES

The lure of Pharaonic Egypt was strong in the Art Deco era, boosted by the discovery in 1922 of Tutankhamen's tomb. Such motifs as stylized wings and dark, exotic eyes, both seen in an ancient wall-painting (*1*), were eagerly adapted by Art Deco jewelers. In the Egyptian taste is a stunning winged-scarab brooch of 1924 by Cartier (*3*), the body of engraved smoked quartz, the wings of faience and diamonds, both dotted with cabochon emeralds. Above that is a similar Cartier design of 1924 for a belt hook (*2*).

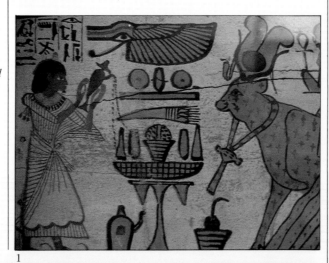

1

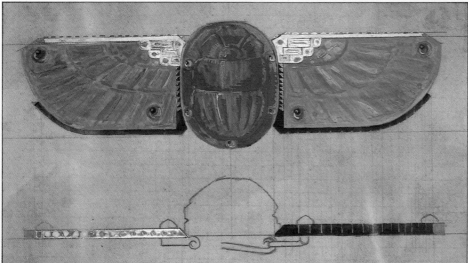

2

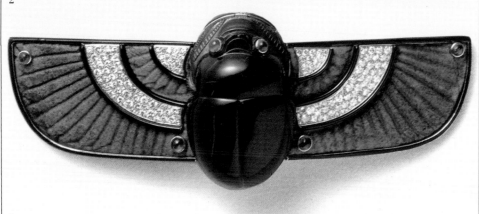

3

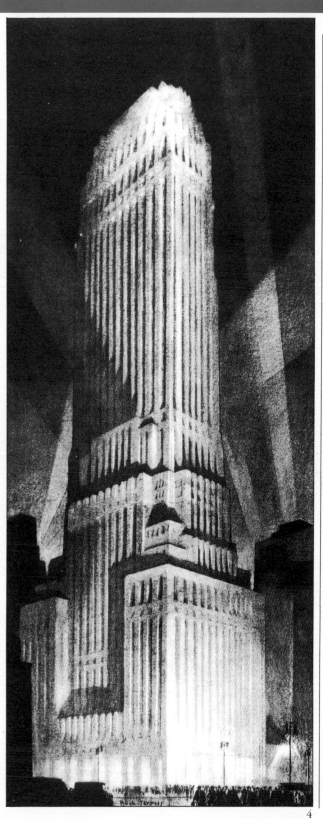

4

The outstanding manifestation of Art Deco in the United States was its architecture: soaring, vertical, stepped, sometimes glittering structures began to define Manhattan's evergrowing skyline. Many of these modern temples of industry were masterpieces of both architecture and interior design, like the Chanin Building (Sloan & Robertson, 1929), seen here in an ethereal period drawing (**4**). Some architectonic jewelry was clearly inspired by such skyscrapers; the stepped clips of gold (**5**) are by Tiffany & Co. of New York.

An interesting correlation between industry and goldsmith's work arose in the Art Deco period: some jewelry designers took their inspiration from the structural make-up of factory machines, metallic behemoths like the Colchester Mascot lathe of the 1920s, a detail of which is illustrated (**7**). Parisian Jean Desprès's silver, silver-gilt, and onyx bracelet (**8**) of 1930, with its crisp silver cabochons and finely turned "hinges," pays distinct homage to the nuts and bolts of the Machine Age. The multi-hued brooch (**6**), probably French, is of white gold set with six cabochon emeralds. A strange configuration of rubies, diamonds, and moonstone completes the design (upside-down, it looks something like an escalator!)

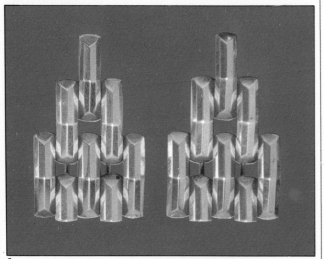

5

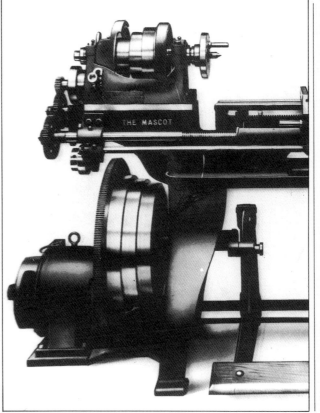

7

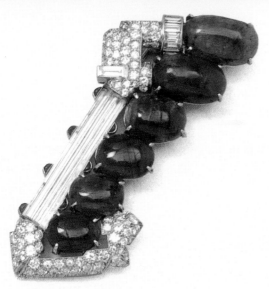

6

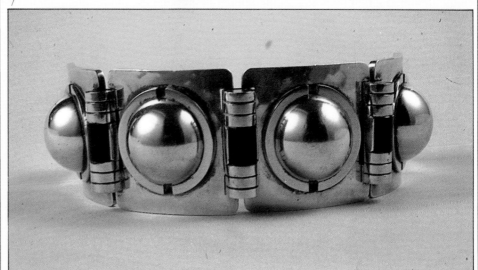

8

PRECIOUS MATERIALS

Precious jewels in the Art Deco period were laden with diamonds, sometimes on their own in blinding masses of icy beauty, sometimes combined with colored precious or even semiprecious stones. A pair of Van Cleef & Arpels drop earrings (1) feature baguette-cut sapphires and pavé-set diamonds. It was Van Cleef that developed the *serti mystérieux*, a setting in which stones are placed next to each other with no visible mount.

The gold and diamond necklace (2) is probably also by Van Cleef & Arpels.

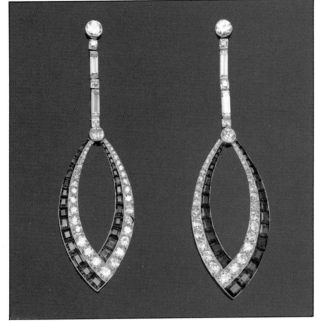

1

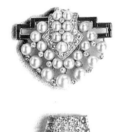

3

4

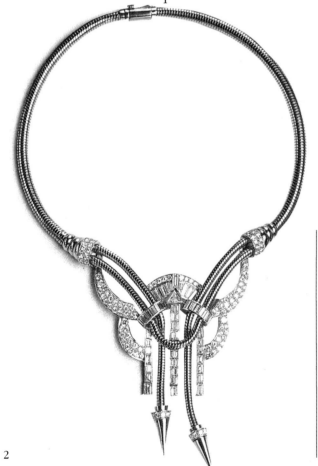

The pearl, diamond and sapphire brooch-clip (3) is by the American firm Marcus & Company, the aquamarine and diamond clips (4), which also form a brooch, by an unknown maker. Clips were an important new fashion accessory in the 1930s, mainly due to their versatility.

The stunning "Stalactite" watch and pendant (5), 1925, is by Cartier; it is set with diamonds, lapis lazuli, an emerald bead, and pearl.

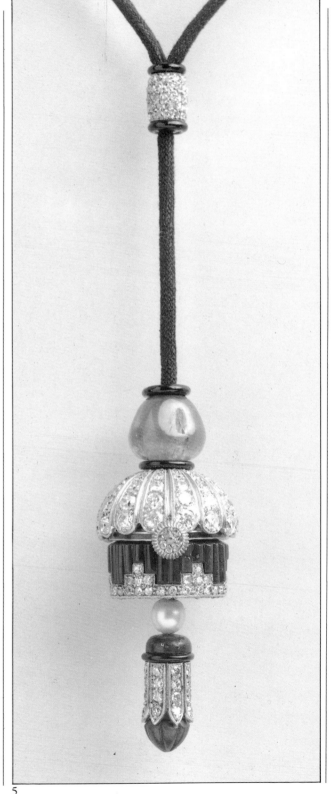

5

2

THE HOUSE OF CARTIER

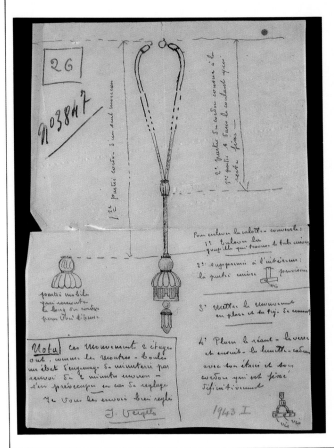

Detailed preliminary design for Cartier's "Stalactite" watch.

Founded in Paris in 1847 by Louis-Francois Cartier, the House of Cartier grew to become one of the world's finest "court jewelers." But it was Louis Cartier (1875–1942), the visionary grandson of the firm's founder, who brought the greatest acclaim to the House of Cartier. His daring, non-traditional designs, and his unabashed love of color and exoticism set him at the forefront of world jewelry design. The year 1910 was a significant one for Cartier: upon viewing the Ballets Russes' production of *Scheherezade,* he and his assistant, Charles Jacqueau, altered not only the firm's palette but also the types of gems they used, opting for semi-precious stones as well as the usual rare gems, sometimes in shocking juxtapositions. Coral, black onyx, diamonds, and

platinum might be combined in one piece, sapphires, emeralds, enamel and gold in another. Motifs both geometric (inspired by Cubist paintings) and Oriental (shaped by trips to the Far East which began in 1908) appeared on Cartier's jewels, as well as floral and figural designs which were subtly stylized in the taste of the day. Besides decorative *bijoux,* timepieces also made up a fair portion of Louis Cartier's output, and in fact he is credited with designing the world's first wristwatch as well as what some consider the most significant wristwatch ever made: the Tank ® watch, inspired by the silhouette of American tanks in the First World War. The arts of China, India, Egypt, and the Islamic world provided a plethora of subjects for the resourceful Cartier, who then took these motifs and absorbed them into the more rectilinear surroundings of Art Deco.

Below is a colorful trio of precious French joaillerie. The Paris jeweler Boucheron created the elaborate cocktail watch (6); it is a sinuous mixture of diamonds, rubies, and platinum. Such ornate timepieces – really bracelets with discreetly hidden watch faces – were highly popular with ladies in the Art Deco period, as were pendant brooches and necklaces with similarly covert timepieces (see the Cartier pendant watch on the previous page). The pendant brooch (7) is made up of diamonds, aquamarines, and a giant citrine; its design is subtly geometric, yet without betraying the traditional roots of its maker, the long-established Parisian firm Maison Mellerio. The maker of the arrow-shaped brooch (8), its diamond body set at one end with a giant emerald drop, at the other with a pearl, is not known.

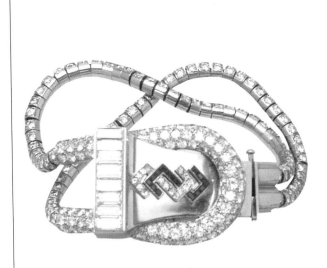

6

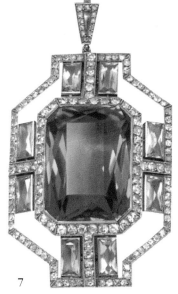

7

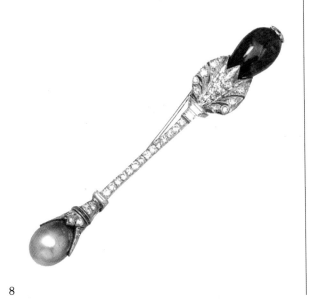

8

STONES

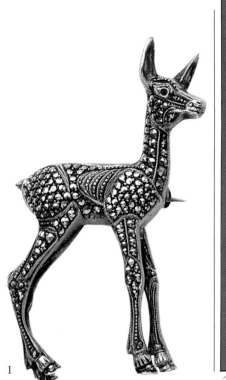

1

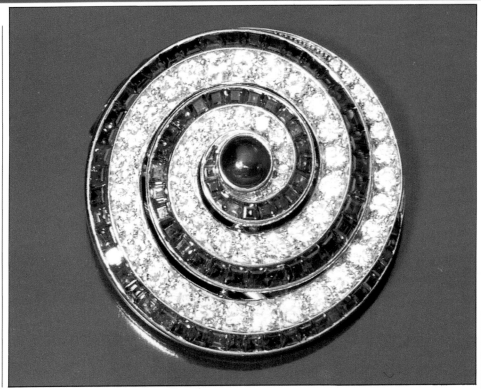

2

From the lowly marcasite to the luxurious baguette-cut diamond – with a rainbow of colorful precious and semiprecious gems (and paste) in between – 1920s and 30s jewelry was rich with stones of every type, cut, and hue. The 1930s silver deer pin (**1**) is set with an array of vari-sized marcasites, their groupings creating interesting patterns on the animal's body. A 1930s Tiffany & Co. brooch (**3**), in the unlikely guise of a swordfish, is made up of diamonds, emeralds, sapphires, and a ruby. The whirling spiral of brilliant-cut diamonds and calibré-cut sapphires around a cabochon sapphire (**2**) was made by the New York jeweler Udall & Ballou.

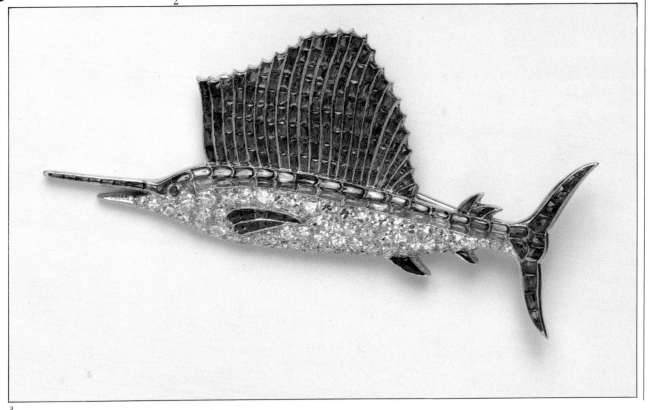

3

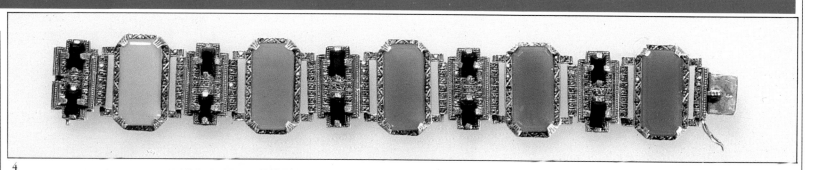

4

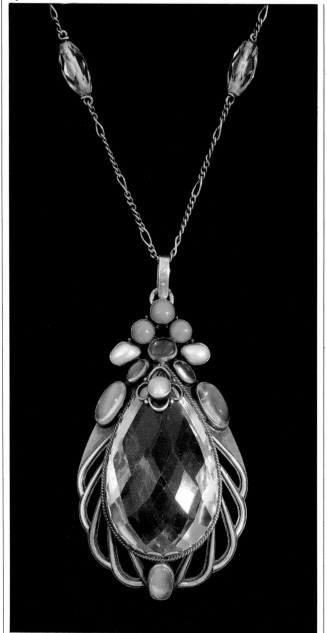

5

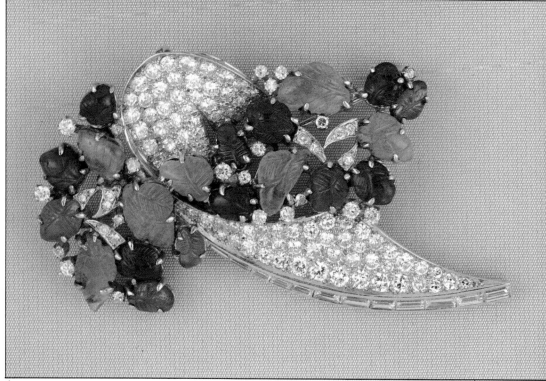

6

The marcasite, chalcedony, and silver bracelet (**4**) with a strong geometric design is from the 1930s; such a piece would have been inexpensive and highly popular. Equally popular, but at the upper end of the price range, was the "fruit salad" or "tutti frutti" type jewel created by the finest joailliers out of diamonds mixed with colorful carved rubies, emeralds, and sapphires. The diamond and platinum cornucopia brooch (**6**) is overflowing with exquisite carved fruit and leaves; it is French, although its maker is unknown. Another rich mélange of stones, this time of the semiprecious variety, is used in the stunning silver necklace and pendant (**5**), set with a teardrop rock crystal, moonstones, pink coral, and pearls. It was handcrafted by H.G. Murphy in the 1920s; Murphy was apprenticed to the English Arts and Crafts metalsmith Henry Wilson, and later set up his own workshop and taught at art colleges. Although this pendant still relates to the Arts and Crafts aesthetic which many designers upheld in 20th-century Britain, it is subtly moderne as well: Murphy was fascinated by the exotic forms of the Ballets Russes, and the rich feather-like composition of this ornate pendant could be considered a nod to Diaghilev and company.

GEOMETRIC SHAPES

The rock crystal, coral, onyx, and sapphire brooch (**1**) is by the firm of the Parisian René Boivin, and is a lovely example of a sparsely geometric, subtly colored jewel. Boivin opened his atelier in 1892; after his death in 1917, his wife, Jeanne (sister of couturier Paul Poiret), and their two daughters took charge of the firm, which continued to thrive well into the 1930s and 40s.

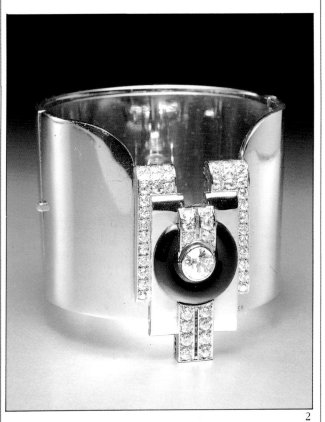

One of Paris's master art-jewelers, Raymond Templier, who worked for the firm founded by his father, Paul, in 1849, produced some of the Art Deco period's boldest geometric designs. The handsome bracelet (**2**), c. 1925–30, is not only a chic, streamlined essay on the circle and the square, but a tour-de-force of ingenuity as well: its central panel, of platinum, white gold, onyx, and diamonds, can be removed and worn as a brooch. The wide bracelet itself is of silver. The cocktail watch by Paul-Emile Brandt (**3**) sports a strong geometric motif on its square-section platinum bracelet, highlighted with diamonds and emeralds; its wide mesh chain is also handsome. Brandt was a Swiss-born jeweler whose career began in the Art Nouveau era, but who later became a respected Art Deco designer.

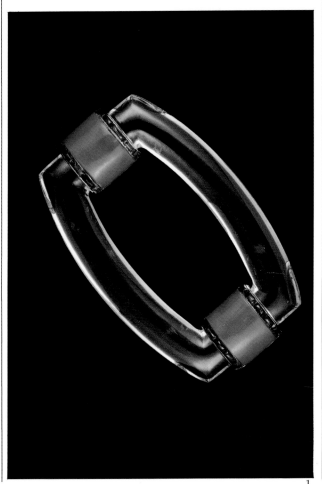

1

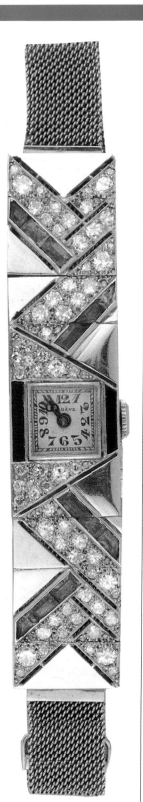

3

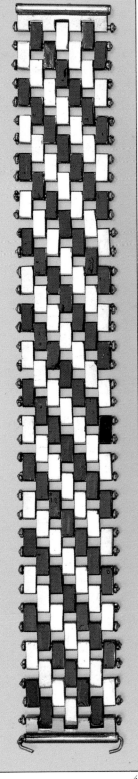

4

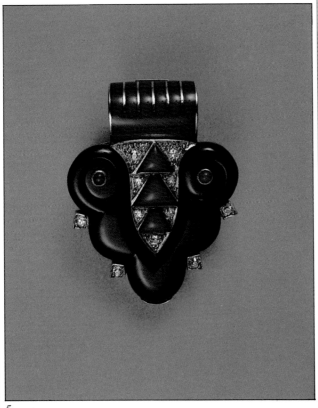

5

Georg Jensen, the Danish silversmith who began making jewelry around the turn of the century, produced this pair of silver clips (**6**) in the 1930s. The two triangles, the smaller superimposed on the larger, are balanced by the addition of the pair of silver balls at their bottom edges. Of course, the clips could be worn pointing up, down, or at any other angle; however they are placed, their strong, simple geometric message is bound to be heard.

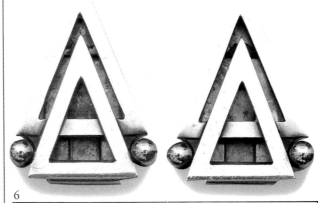

6

The wide, multi-linked bracelet (**4**), with its continuous diagonal motif, is made of enameled and silvered white metal. This wholly geometric French costume jewel dates from the 1930s; its design echoes those of similar bracelets in gold of the same period. The red-enameled and subtly voluted geometric elements on the gold, onyx, and diamond clip by Cartier (**5**) seem secondary to its overall billowy shape. The strict symmetry and primary color scheme of this unusual piece make it a most striking Art Deco jewel.

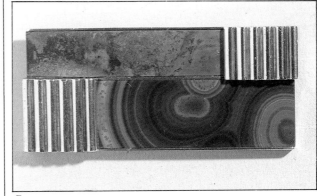

7

The silver, malachite, and sodalite brooch (**7**) was made in the 1930s by Jean Desprès, whose works betray his industrial-design training during the First World War. The Parisian master has combined four simple elements of metal and stone and come up with a bold essay in surface and texture. The silk-smooth but deeply mottled surfaces of the semiprecious blue and green stones contrast strongly with the monochromatic but ridged silver.

DECO MOTIFS

Although today's images of the Jazz Age are dominated by frilly flappers and tuxedoed gentlemen, the types of figures appearing on Art Deco jewels ranged from the Neo-classical to the moderne. The modishly dressed lady walking her equally elegant borzoi (**1**), a yellow-metal brooch, is probably English and from the 1930s.

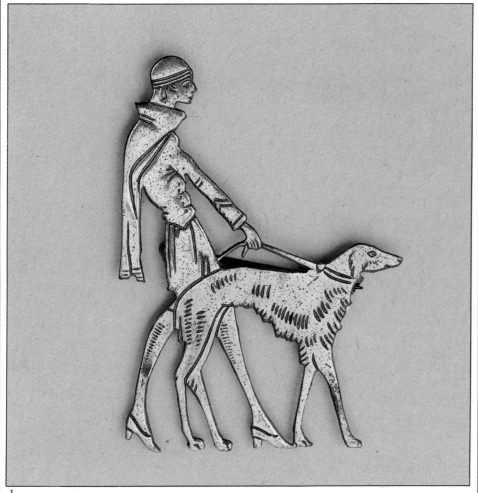

1

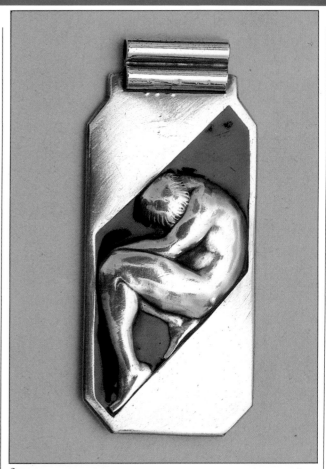

2

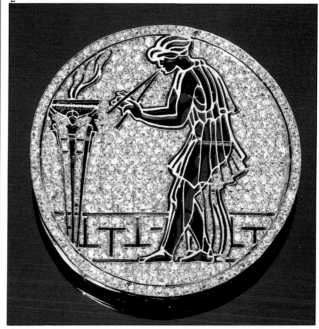

3

The handsome 1920s enameled-silver pendant (**2**), its monumental male nude a zigzag of flesh confined within a parallelogram-like space, is by the Frenchman Emile Davide. Another traditional figure, but this one lyrical and light, is the Arcadian pipe-player occupying the roundel of pavé-set diamonds (**3**); this brooch is by Boucheron and dates from the 1910s.

Oriental motifs, and the stylized sunburst frequently appeared on both precious and costume jewels of the 1920s and 30s. On a bracelet from Marsh & Co. of San Francisco (**4**) carved-coral bird and plant plaques alternate with ideograms of iron. The pendant in the form of a pagoda (**5**) is by the German firm Theodor Fahrner.

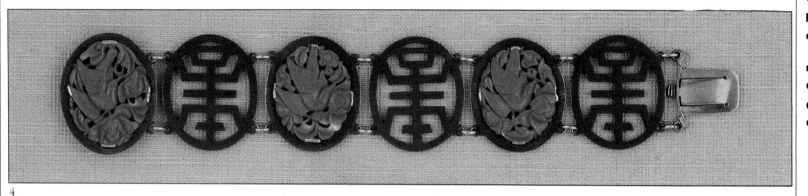

4

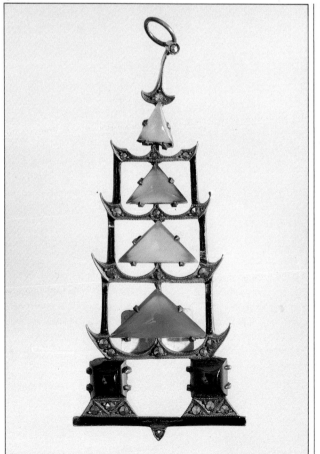

5

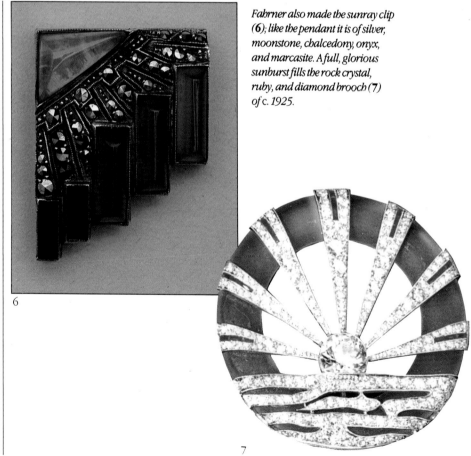

6

Fahrner also made the sunray clip (**6**); like the pendant it is of silver, moonstone, chalcedony, onyx, and marcasite. A full, glorious sunburst fills the rock crystal, ruby, and diamond brooch (**7**) of c. 1925.

7

NEW MATERIALS

Synthetic plastics breathed colorful new life into the costume jewelry industry in the 20th century, as this richly hued quartet of clips and brooches (**2**) shows. Plastic was in fact a mid-19th-century invention: the British scientist Alexander Parkes produced cellulose nitrate, or, as he called it, Parkesine, in 1855. Since then, an ever-improving range of substances – opaque, translucent, mottled, marbled, variously molded – have appeared as rings, clips, brooches, bracelets, and necklaces.

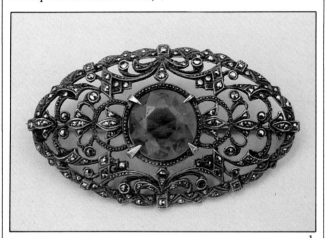

1

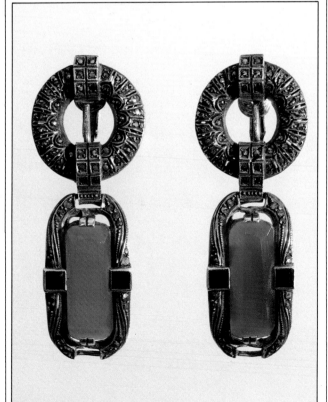

2

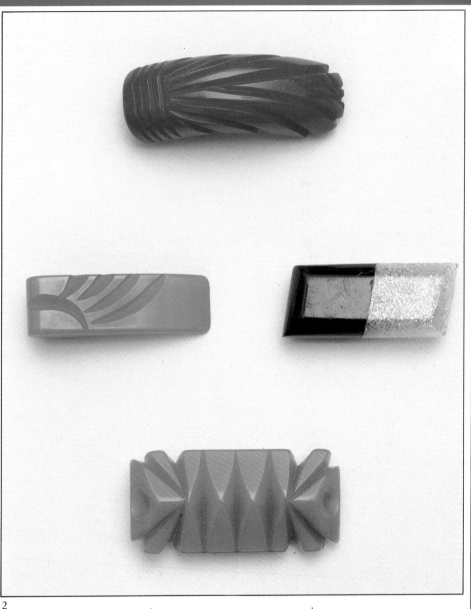

3

This silver, marcasite, and paste brooch (**1**) has a busy, quasi-organic quality, although it dates from the 1920s or 30s: some European costume jewelry at this time still bore vestigial Victorian or Art Nouveau motifs. On the other hand, the hanging earrings of silver, marcasite, carnelian, and onyx (**3**) have a much more period feel, with their geometric composition; they were made at Theodor Fahrner's Pforzheim factory in the mid-1920s. Cut-steel studs and marcasites are often confused; the latter, in fact, are cut from iron pyrites, which have a highly reflective surface and hence make good diamond substitutes. Both cut steel and marcasite began to be used for jewelry in the late 1700s, with marcasite coming into vogue again in the 1920s.

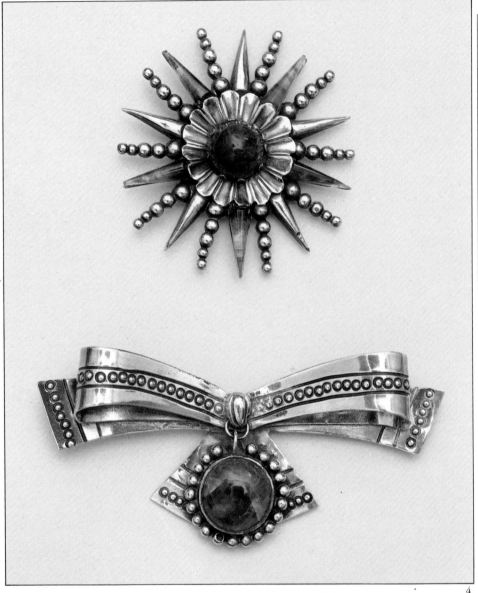

From an unlikely source came a range of handsome bijoux in the 1930s: American architect/designer William Spratling, who settled in Taxco, Mexico, in 1929, produced an array of dramatic jewels, including the floriform and beribboned brooches (4), of silver and amethyst. The origin of the handsome Bakelite and chrome necklace (5) is unknown, but it is probably French or German. Its chrome mesh chain is especially handsome, as are its repeated circular motifs.

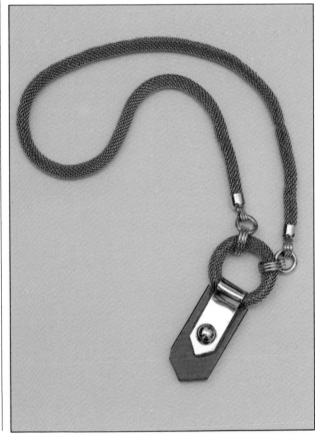

4

5

Bracelets and bangles of plastic and new metal combinations appeared in huge numbers in the 1920s and 30s, and flappers liked to wear them en masse, snaking all the way up their arms. The Bakelite bangle (6), one of its two parts molded to a subtle point, is French, and the nickel-plated-metal expanding bracelet (7), with its Machine Age overtones, is possibly American; both are from the 1930s.

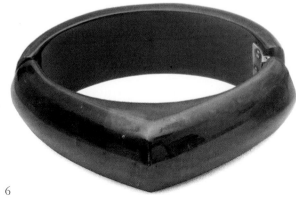

6

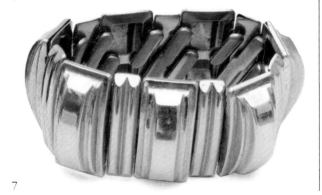

7

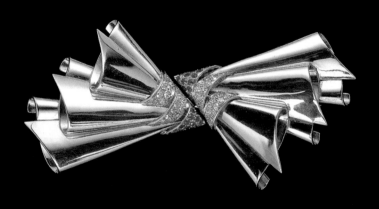

A 1940s double-clip brooch in gold, rubies, and diamonds.

CHAPTER EIGHT

THE POSTWAR PERIOD

1940-1959

The war legacy

·

The Surrealists

·

Costume jewelry

VIVIENNE BECKER

INTRODUCTION

Jewelry of the 1940s is sometimes called cocktail jewelry, – appropriately, because it is very much a lively cocktail of 20th-century themes and inspirations. The style evolved from the tail end of Art Deco design, but exuded a robust energy and assertiveness of its own. In the midst of the gloom of World War II, jewelry was bursting with red gold and rubies, ribbons of yellow gold, and showers of sapphires, substantial chunks of citrines, aquamarines, and amethysts, and huge, plump drop-shaped moonstones.

Ingredients of the basic cocktail design were taken from various aspects of Art Deco and the Machine Age. In the 1940s the streamlined, stark architectural lines of modernist jewels were softened into more voluptuous curves, inflated into massive, three-dimensional shapes, and coaxed into figurative forms. One of the most striking features of this design is the successful mixture of opposing elements: motifs that are both natural and unnatural, stiff and fluid, static yet full of movement. Early cocktail jewels of the late 1930s or early 1940s still looked geometric and abstract, like bulkier versions of Art Deco pieces; as the decade wore on, they became softer, more full of color and movement and texture.

Machinery in motion became the most dominant influence on jewels of the 1940s. There was an obsessive interest in tools, machines, how they worked and moved, which manifested itself in jewel design as motifs of screw heads, ball bearings, girders, rods, in metalwork constructed like flexible brickwork or tire tracks, all reminiscent of the rhythm of the assembly line or a moving staircase.

Cocktail Jewelry

Cocktail jewelry was bred in an atmosphere of enormous change and crisis, of social, economic, and political upheaval. Two world wars had brought a drastic redistribution of wealth, and women had now won a good measure of independence and authority. The new breed of working women created a market for fashionable ready-to-wear clothes and accessories, while financial difficulties also forced some wealthy customers to make economies without sacrificing style or outward confidence. However grim their everyday lives, most women went to the cinema and were exposed, first-hand, to all the glamour of Hollywood. Glamour and escapism was much in demand in the 1940s, yet there was simply not the same amount of money to spend on masses of diamonds and platinum. Instead, to achieve the effect of massive magnificence, limited quantities of gold were eked out and cleverly wrought to look like heavy chunks of sumptuous metal. Gold was often stamped out from thin sheets to give the effect of substantial weight.

As sleek geometry gave way to sculptural forms, there was a move toward the use of wide expanses of sweeping metal, rose pink gold, or rich yellow-gold, wrought into

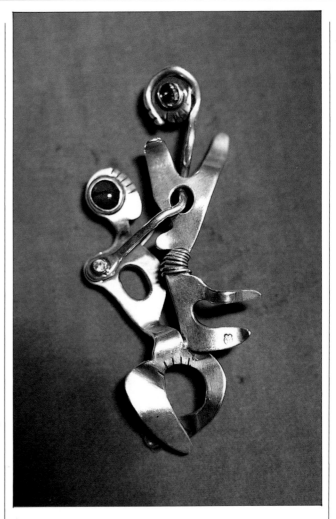

gauche swirls, whorls, drapes. In contrast to the chic black and white of the mid-1920s, color became all-important, integrated by the use of colored gold and transparent semi-precious stones. Metal was textured for added interest: a pattern of perforated hexagons, creating a honeycomb design, was a favorite feature of Van Cleef & Arpels in the 1940s, or little overlapping semicircles like shiny scales. Gold mesh, imitating gauze or lattice and basketwork, became especially popular in the late 1940s and 1950s. Fabric motifs predominated, and gold looked like drapes, bows, knots, with added bouncy movement of tassels or bobbles.

In contrast to the static geometry of Art Deco, movement became the central feature of cocktail jewelry design. There was a contrived stiffness to the pleats and folds and drapes of cocktail jewels, but the overall effect was one of wild movement and flexibility. Chain was often ribbed or folded like an accordian in a style known as gas pipe, for obvious reasons, or it could be knitted into a tight mesh rope of herringbone pattern, or bouncy spring like coils.

The air of unreality that touched the 1920s and 30s still affected the ever-popular flower jewels of the 1940s and 50s. Gold and gem-set blossoms were made like naive, shiny buttercups or stiff, star-shaped flowers. Van Cleef & Arpels produced the most spectacular flowers of the period, using their new invisible settings, in which masses of tiny, square-cut rubies or sapphires were held from behind by a gold framework only, so that no means of setting could be seen from the front.

Amusing figurative motifs, and cartoon-like animals gradually crept into jewel design in the mid-1940s. There were stiff childlike figures of scarecrows, clowns, gardeners or flower-sellers and, most characteristic of all, the ballerina, set with tiny colored gems. The range of amusing figures and animals was one aspect that continued into the 1950s. It was Cartier, and particularly the designer Jeanne Toussaint, who helped build up the fashion for fantasy creatures, for perky animal and bird of paradise jewels. The big cats, the panthers and leopards, that have become the luxurious but poignant symbols of the Duchess of Windsor, were perfected in Cartier's workshops in the 1940s and 50s.

The Second World War in Europe had depleted the jewelry-making industry. Jewelers' premises had been destroyed, and many of the skilled workforce had left to join the army or were co-opted into war work, as jewelers were well equipped to undertake precision engineering. Cartier's craftsmen, for example, spent the war making camera parts and navigational equipment. Jewelers who did manage to continue in business found precious metals and stones scarce – sometimes even unobtainable. However, with the liberation of Paris in October 1944, the great names – Boucheron, Cartier, Chaumet, and Van Cleef & Arpels – were able to open for business again.

The boldness of 1940s jewelry belonged to the major grand-jewels houses, the leaders in the field. Van Cleef & Arpels, Boucheron, Chaumet, Lacloche, Mauboussin, Mellerio and their neighbours in and around the Place Vendôme all excelled in the cocktail style. As the influence of war was less pervasive in the United States, American jewelers or New York branches of Parisian houses flourished at this time – in particular, Paul Flato, John Rubel, Verdura, Traebert and Hoeffer. In Italy, Bulgari led a band of jewelers working in the cocktail mood, and in Switzerland major watch firms produced stylish cocktail wristwatches, popular accessories of the period. In England, trade was slowly resumed after the war, and the prevailing style in Europe was adopted gradually by London manufacturers such as D. Shackman and Byworth.

Newly liberated from the deprivation of wartime, the designers of costume jewelery felt free to experiment, making pieces out of gold-plated base metals, silver gilt,

and paste which were hard to distinguish from those worth one hundred times as much. Costume jewelry design even began to influence those who worked in traditional precious metals and stones.

The Fashionable Fifties

As with most ages, during the 1950s, there was a two-tier system of jewelry: expensive gem-set pieces, made by famous jewelry houses, in mainstream fashions; or the artist-craftsman's jewelry, made in smaller workshops from less expensive materials, in which design and artistic spirit were the most important elements.

In expensive jewelry, a sophisticated all-white, all-diamond look predominated. The emphasis in design was on movement, and to achieve this soignée effect, diamonds of different cuts and shapes were used together to create, swirls, twirls, fans, waterfalls and cascades. The little rod-shaped baguette diamond, beloved of the Art Deco jewelers, was enormously popular once again, but was now incorporated into far more voluptuous, curvaceous patterns. Huge, majestic flower sprays were also typical of the late 1940s and 50s, politely luscious,

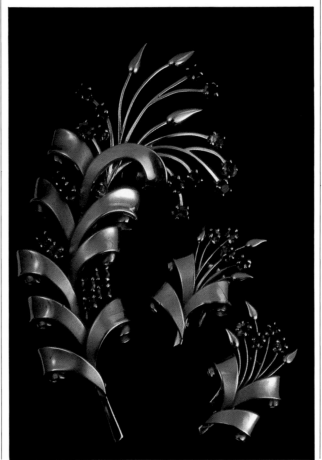

This gold brooch and earring set combines two distinct styles; the chunkiness of 40s cocktail jewelry in the ribbon-like curls of the leaves, with the much lighter and more delicate spray-forms that could be found dotting many a lapel in the 1950s. The transition from the lightly contained designs of the 30s, through the beginnings of movement in the coctail jewelry of the 40s to the light swirls and open forms in the 50s, reflected a decisive change of mood among designers – a mood caught from society in general which was wanting new and "modern" designs.

INTRODUCTION

extravagant blooms, their petals pavé set with diamonds or colored gems, mixed often with butter-yellow gold which was increasingly popular from the late 1930s through the 1940s and 50s. A combination of gold filigree wire or lattice openwork, with diamonds was popular around 1950, concocted into stylized flower sprays with the dynamic movement of the 1940s and the icy sophistication of the 1950s.

Alongside the traditional, majestic white diamond look, expensive jewelry in the 1950s featured coral and tur-

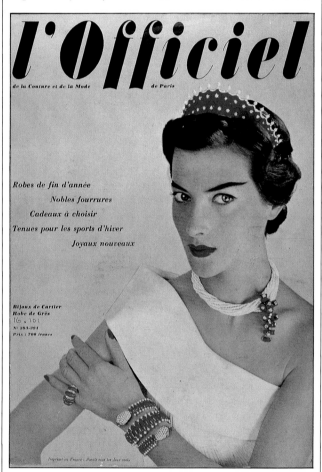

quoise, mixed with flounces of bristling yellow gold and scatterings of diamonds. Some abstract designs heralded the new organic mood of the 1960s; others were based on cocktail age flowers, birds insects. The coral ladybug, alone or poised on a gold flower or leaf, its body set with tiny diamonds, enriched with enamels perhaps, onyx, or lapis lazuli, was a hallmark of 1950s jewelry design and a favorite motif at Cartier. Starfish jewels were worn in the 1950s, in gold and diamonds or perhaps with smooth coral tentacles, while shells and seahorses illustrated the mystery and magic of the ocean. Birds and animals in many cases

also became more fantastic, the static quality of 1940s designs giving way to extra vitality and a sense of soaring movement, particularly in the design of sweeping tail feathers, wings stretched backward against the wind, and quirky inquisitive heads pointed toward the light. Pierre Sterlé in Paris was the champion of this style of the 1950s. He used an almost baroque combination of colored gems, precious and semiprecious, mixing amethysts with turquoises for example, and generously adding fringes of gold mesh or chain, gold textured wings, or feathers, enlivened with showers of diamonds.

Fine Art

A number of prominent painters and sculptors moved into jewelry-making as a new area of artistic expression. The first of these were the Swiss sculptor Alberto Giacometti and the American sculptor, best known for his mobiles, Alexander Calder. Ernst, Cocteau, de Chirico, Man Ray, Tanguy, and Dubuffet followed, each of whom produced small collections.

By the early 1960s, Georges Braque had designed more than 130 pieces which were exhibited in the Musée des Arts Décoratifs in Paris. These featured Braque's unique interpretation of mythological scenes, and were often made in textured gold superimposed on slabs of cut stone, rhodocrosite, or lapis lazuli.

Even more prolific was the Spanish surrealist, Salvador Dali. He produced a large collection of surreal pieces – soft watches, a cross of gold sugar lumps, an enameled platinum eye with a jeweled tear dripping, a golden heart containing a sack of pulsating rubies, an elephant with spider's legs. Many of these pieces were unwearable, but Dali claimed his work was in the tradition of Benvenuto Cellini, Sandro Botticelli, and Leonardi da Vinci. He also claimed that his work encompassed "physics, mathematics, architecture, nuclear science; the pyscho-nuclear, the mystico-nuclear" and that it was "a protest against emphasis on the cost of the materials of jewelry." In these aims, he was anticipating much of the contemporary approach.

In Italy, other fine artists began to get involved in jewelry. The first was the sculptor Bruno Martinazzi. Many of his pieces are strongly sculptural, with an emphasis on texture. He builds his designs layer by layer, often incorporating different-colored golds and even platinum in a single piece. Gemstones – usually diamonds – are pavé-set as highlights. He was followed by the Pomodoro brothers – Arnaldo, a sculptor and architect, and Gio, a painter and graphic designer – whose work has a more deliberate, planned quality, almost as if incorporating other disciplines into their jewelry work.

In Germany, aeronautical engineer Friedrick Becker turned professional goldsmith in 1947 and brought with him an aesthetic built on machine engineering and aerospace technology. His pieces are composed of polished, geometric forms, sometimes even with moving parts.

Democratic Designs

As far as less expensive jewelry was concerned in the 1950s, there was an exciting move toward 'modern' artistic silver jewels, very much in tune with the generally rather austere style of the decorative arts. Silver suited the smooth, floating lines characteristic of Fifties designs in general. Its subtle tones and textures were perfect for capturing organic designs, the spindly Calder-inspired spirals, but at the same time they were strong enough to interpret the sharp, zigzag motifs of the oncoming electronic age –the "electrocardiogram" element of Fifties design.

From the 1930s, Scandinavian jewelers often used the simple shapes they derived from folk art to produce new "democratic" designs. These deliberately avoided the over-ornamentation which other European jewelers used to impress their noble clientele. The smooth, clean lines and reverence for natural materials that typified the Scandinavian approach found itself in the ascendancy in a postwar period in which the grip of social class had been eroded. As the style was refined it became a growing influence on other European designers.

The early exponent of the Scandinavian style was Georg Jensen. Trained as a sculptor, he specialized in a distinctive, sculptural style, almost always figurative or organic, but highly stylized and precise. Jensen died in 1935, but his Copenhagen-based company became a major influence after the war. The firm's enlightened artistic policy was maintained by Jensen's son, Soren Georg Jensen. Hanna Ditzel, the architectural designer, has worked for Jensen since 1954, and a host of other famous names designed for the firm – Herlow, Koppel, Malinowski, Mohl-Hansen, Pedersen and Rohde. Henning Koppel's designs for Jensen are among the most distinctive of the age.

In America, the industry was less affected by the war, and started off the postwar period with an exhibition in 1946 in New York's Museum of Modern Art, where some 135 pieces were exhibited by 46 artists. Two years later, twice as many artists exhibited at Minneapolis's Walker Art Center, and in 1955 a Museum of Contemporary Crafts was founded in New York. In 1960, the US Government established the American Crafts Council, which opened regional centers throughout the country where craftsmen could hold seminars, workshops, and exhibitions.

But America did not have only the seed corn of its own native talent to depend on. It was awash with hundreds of European artists and jewelers, forced out of Europe by the war and bringing with them the influence of the Bauhaus. In 1940, Margaret de Patta began studying under Lazlo Moholy-Nagy, first at a summer school, then at the School of Design in Chicago that he had set up. Influenced by

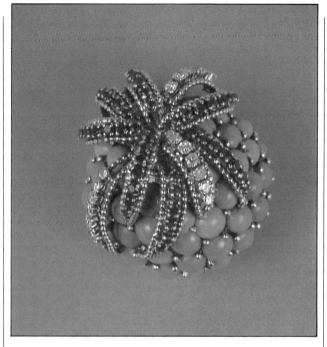

Picasso, she created miniature silver sculptures, and became an influential figure in American jewelry with her bold use of new materials and techniques.

The Bauhaus ideology of breaking with all traditional restraints found fertile soil in the USA. Sam Kramer began incorporating *objets trouvés* (found objects) in his jewelry, aping other contemporary American fine artists who were using the sculptural and painterly technique of assemblage. These works further eroded the barriers between jewelry and sculpture. He even anticipated the 1960s by drawing inspiration from science fiction comics.

Kramer's shop in New York's Greenwich Village encouraged others. Harlem-born black artist Arthur Smith moved to Greenwich Village in the 1940s and began to produce large neckpieces and bracelets intended to be body adornments rather than simple fashion accessories. These too anticipated the revolution in jewelry that was to come about in the 1960s.

The established companies who still produce luxury goods have seen no need to experiment with new design concepts. Much of their work relies on classic jewelry forms, exquisitely fabricated and set with flawless gems, like the piece from Van Cleef & Arpels (late 1950s-60s)). It is set with rubies, turquoises, and diamonds – with organic imagery in evidence – but there is no attempt at realism. This jewelry is for a world of glamor, set apart from the harsh realities of life.

151

INFLUENCES

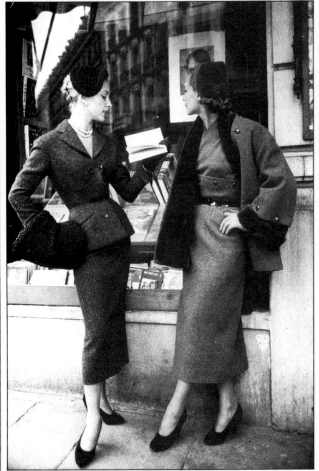

1

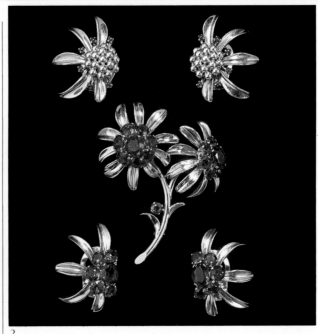

2

Paris resumed the lead in couture fashion after the Second World War. Styles retained their simplicity, but indicated a move away from frugality with longer skirts and more attention to detail. These tweed suits from Balmain (**1**), illustrated in the British magazine Picture Post in 1953, show feminine nipped-in waists and more complex pattern-cutting than would have been considered sensible in the war years. Jewelry was worn as another mere detail. Small, pretty brooch and earring sets, such as the gold and citrine set in the bottom of the picture (**2**), were popular for everyday wear. Flowers were an endless source of design inspiration during the 1950s.

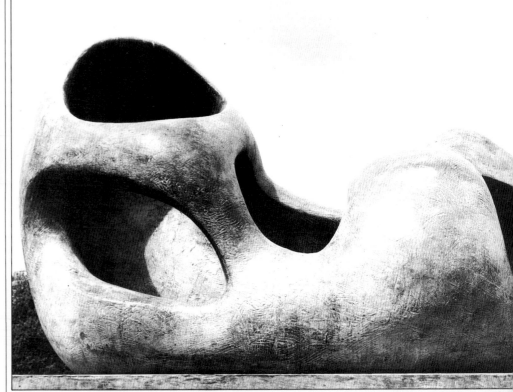

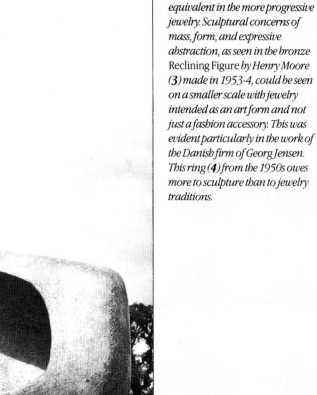

4

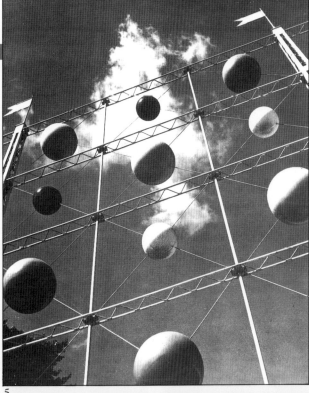

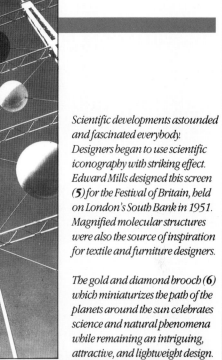

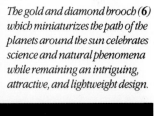

5

Scientific developments astounded and fascinated everybody. Designers began to use scientific iconography with striking effect. Edward Mills designed this screen (5) for the Festival of Britain, held on London's South Bank in 1951. Magnified molecular structures were also the source of inspiration for textile and furniture designers.

The gold and diamond brooch (6) which miniaturizes the path of the planets around the sun celebrates science and natural phenomena while remaining an intriguing, attractive, and lightweight design.

Developments in fine art had their equivalent in the more progressive jewelry. Sculptural concerns of mass, form, and expressive abstraction, as seen in the bronze Reclining Figure by Henry Moore (3) made in 1953-4, could be seen on a smaller scale with jewelry intended as an art form and not just a fashion accessory. This was evident particularly in the work of the Danish firm of Georg Jensen. This ring (4) from the 1950s owes more to sculpture than to jewelry traditions.

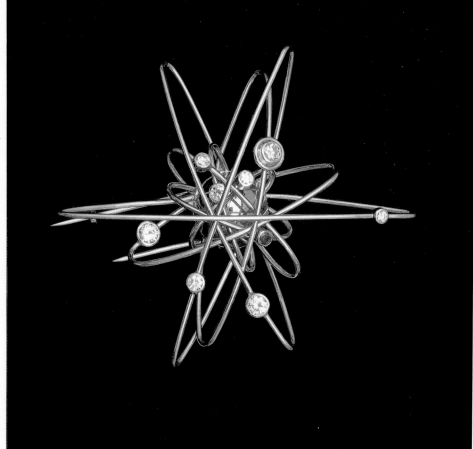

3

6

TRADITIONAL LUXURY

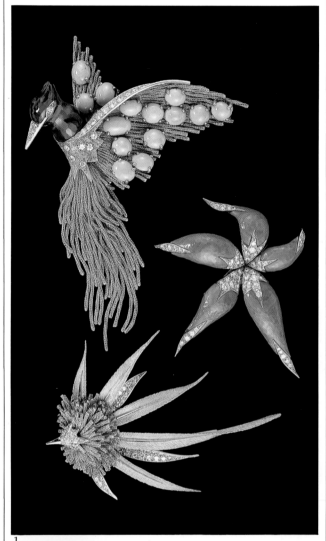

Colorful and exotic images caught the imagination of Europeans still experiencing the austerity of the war years. These three brooches (**1**) from Sterle of Paris in the 1940s capture the natural sweeping asymmetry of flora and fauna, something not seen in the more constrained Art Deco designs. They seem to symbolize freedom and romanticism, transporting the imagination to tropical gardens of a mysterious underwater world.

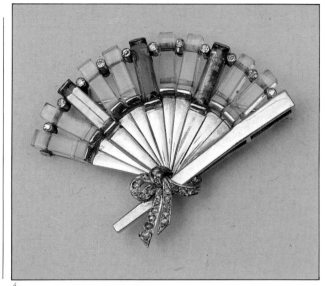

Despite its passage into public ownership in the 1960s, the firm of Cartier still dominates the world of luxury jewelry. The famous series of leopard and panther jewelry remains as sought after today as ever, as the sale of this sapphire and diamond panther clip (**3**) from the Duchess of Windsor's collection testifies. Made by Cartier in 1949, the panther is pavé-set with diamonds and caliber-cut sapphire spots with pear-shaped yellow diamond eyes. It is crouching on a large cabochon sapphire.

The older firms famous for their exquisite gem-set jewelry tend to stay with more traditional designs. Another family firm from Paris, Boucheron, produced this fan-shaped brooch (**4**) in the 1950s. With its Oriental prettiness it could easily have adorned a genteel Victorian lady; nothing in its design would place it in the 20th century.

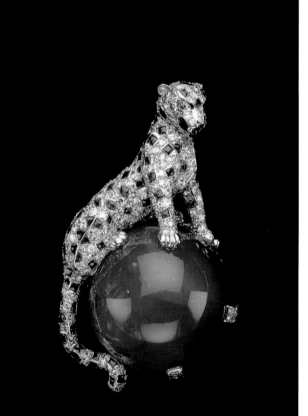

Jewelers returned to more literal translations of flowers, birds, and animals in the 1940s and 50s. The mushroom brooch (**2**), possibly by Van Cleef & Arpels, appears charmingly naïve. The stalks illustrate a trend toward the use of wire as a means of creating surface texture and lightening the weight of jewelry, both visually and physically.

The restrictions of 1937 did not prevent Van Cleef & Arpels from producing this sumptuous Jarretière bracelet (**6**). To aid the reflective quality of the gems the cushion-shaped sapphires and baguette diamonds are invisibly set – a technique invented by the maker. The ring is by the American "King of Diamonds," Harry Winston. He bought the diamond, in the collection of Washington hostess Evalyn Walsh McClean, in 1940 and sold it the following year to the Duke and Duchess of Windsor.

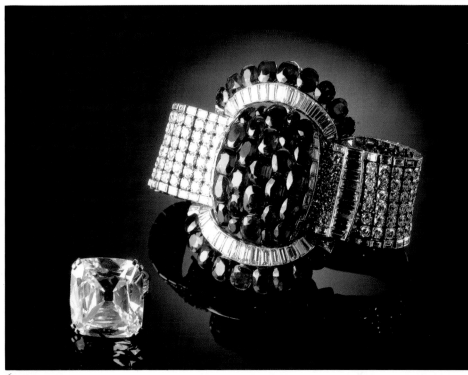

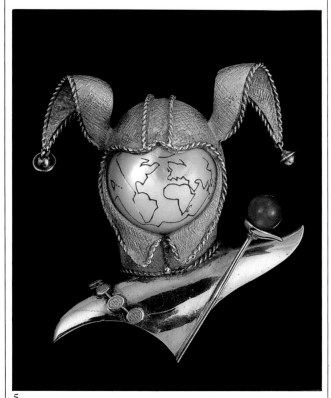

5

The Paris family firm of Chaumet specialized in tiaras and jeweled liveries for Indian potentates. Like other famous companies they cultivated the custom of royal families around the world, which may explain the mother-of-pearl globe in their brooch "Le Spectacle du Monde" (**5**), of the late 1950s60s, but not its surrealistic setting in a jester's hat.

The styles of the younger jewelers who started out at the end of the 1950s can be easily distinguished. Since 1954, De Beers has organized the annual Diamonds International awards, which both encourage new jewelers to be innovative and give them publicity. The rings (**7**) are four British winners from the early 1960s: left, John Donald; center top, Geoffrey Turk; center bottom, Podolsky; right, David Thomas.

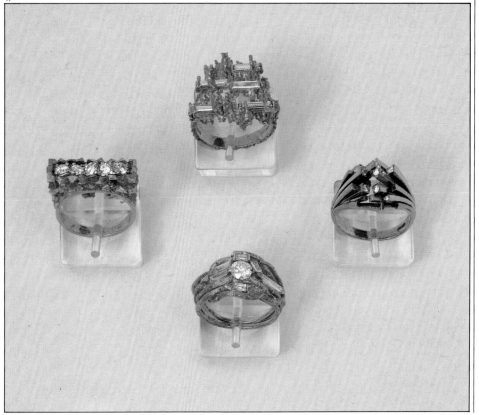

EVERYDAY ACCESSORIES

The smart tailored suits worn by women in the 1950s provided an excellent background for brightly colored, cheerful-looking jewelry. Neat brooches, often worn on the lapel of a coat or jacket, were popular everyday wear. The enameled silver basket of flowers from the 1950s (**1**) is a timeless and nostalgic reminder of the pastoral idyll close to the heart of many a city worker. Many more women were earning a wage by this time and able to buy good-quality costume jewelry.

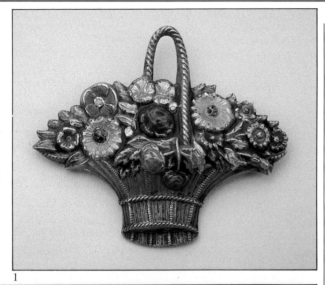

1

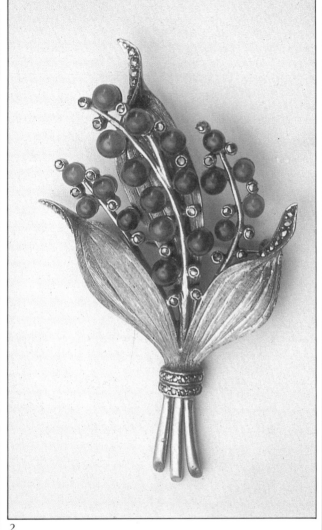

2

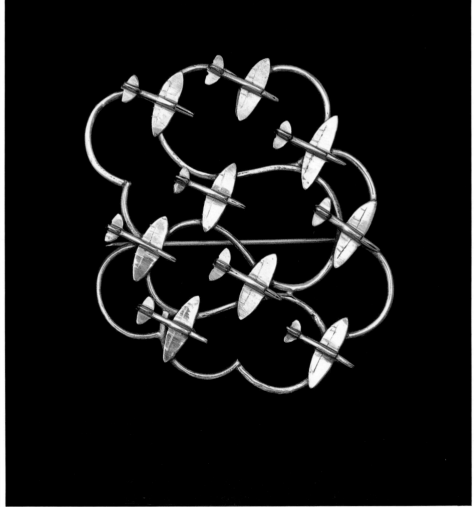

3

Gently swaying floral sprays again lent color and an interesting curvaceous form to brooches in the 1950s. This example in silver gilt and chrysoprase (**2**) is typical of the period. The emotive use of bunches of flowers created a feeling of joie de vivre and romanticism, very aptly coinciding, in Britain, with the end of rationing and utility product designs.

Wartime images were still fresh in everybody's memory. A formation of little silver airplanes sweeping across a female chest shows a fair degree of humor (**3**), but no doubt it also held deeper significance for the wearer. It was quite common for military insignia and miniature hardware, like boats and planes, to appear in jewelry during the war.

By the 1940s and 50s costume jewelry was rivaling the real thing. Improved technology in casting, plating, and creating paste gems made better quality "fakes" a feasible alternative to gold and gemstones (see **5**). The glamor of the Hollywood movie stars and wealthy socialites could now be emulated by the middle class woman, helped by good ready-to-wear copies of couture clothing and skillfully produced costume jewelry.

Many more people had the money and time to entertain, as well as the chance to look spectacular at an affordable price, and so the era of the cocktail party (originally just a pursuit of the wealthy), took off. Cocktail jewelry was very popular, and its chunkiness lent itself to costume copies. Art Deco imagery was still evident, but more fun and movement came in with bows and swirls and folds (**4**). The popularity of costume jewelry made the market dynamic and competitive. Designers could be freer and less conservative, and in many ways left the traditional jewelers lagging behind.

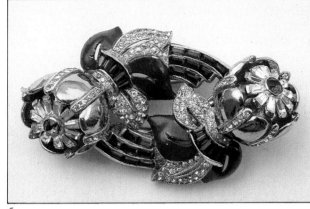

5

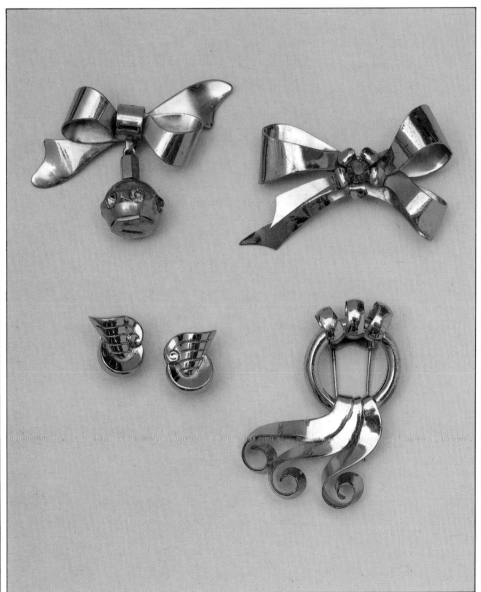

4

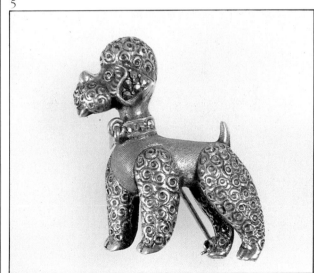

6

Witty images like the marcasite French poodle brooch (**6**) were used to make the business-like tailored suit more fun. Animals shaped like Walt Disney cartoon characters and resplendent birds of paradise signified the wish for a brighter and less troubled future.

ABSTRACT INNOVATORS

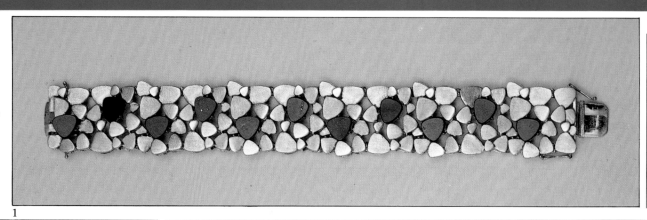

The northern European move away from the glitz of burnished gold and diamonds can be seen in this white gold and lapis lazuli bracelet (**1**) from Amsterdam in the 1950s. The surface decoration is provided by the slight change in height and angle of the segments. With its machine-like finish, the piece appeals through its subtle simplicity and precision.

1

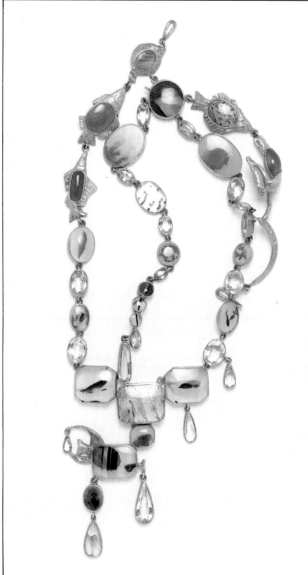

2

MARGARET DE PATTA (1903-64)

The term "artist jeweler" came into its own in the 1970s, but those who pioneered the concept can be picked out from much earlier. Margaret de Patta was one of them. She studied painting and sculpture at the Academy of Fine Arts in San Diego (1921-23), the California School of Fine Arts in San Francisco (1923-25), and the Art Students League in New York (1926-29). Without losing her artistic intentions, she turned her attention to jewelry in 1929. To be free from craft traditions and technical limitations she studied and mastered many jewelry skills.

A summer school in 1940, run by the ex-Bauhaus artist Lazlo Moholy-Nagy, had a significant effect on her development. Bauhaus ideas reinforced the

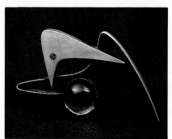

De Patta's 1947 silver and quartz crystal brooch reflects her interest in expressive artforms, which grew from her early training as a painter and sculptor.

validity of her experimental methods: counter to the traditions of the time, she used such materials as stainless steel and plastic in her work, and in 1941 she collaborated with the lapidary Francis J. Sperisen,

exploring the reflective qualities of stones with new cuts. Her work was so well received that in 1946 she began to produce prototypes for manufacture. Her jewelry proved to be a successful competitor to costume jewelry, but she never lost sight of her original aim to create expressive artforms with her jewelry.

Margaret de Patta was generous in her encouragement of other jewelers, teaching and lecturing until her death, and was active in the promotion and development of jewelry via the Metal Arts Guild, Designer Craftsmen in California, and the American Crafts Council.

"Individuality," the watchword of the 1970s, has never been totally absent from jewelry. This necklace (**2**) is by Sah Oved, second daughter of a country doctor, and born in 1900 as Gwendolen Ethel Rendle. She found a rich source of

inspiration for her work when she met Mosheh Oved. He was a Polish Jew whose culture and folklore strongly influenced Sah's work. Cameo Corner, his shop on London's Museum Street, provided a treasure chest of raw materials

for her highly original pieces. She decided early in her life to be a jeweler, but worked with little formal training. Finally she studied silversmithing at the Central School of Arts and Crafts, London, during the 1950s.

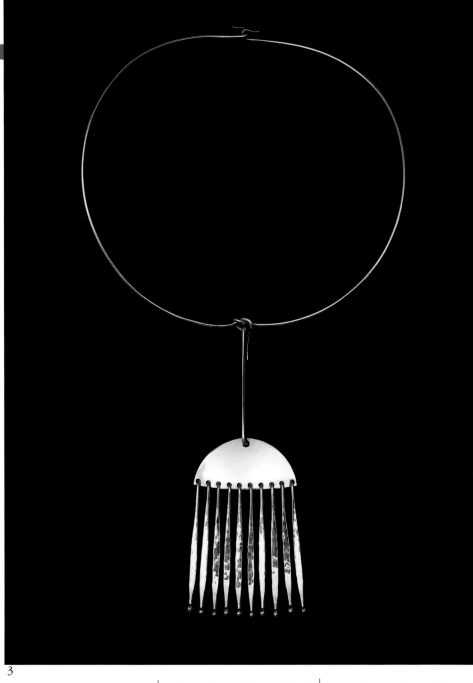

3

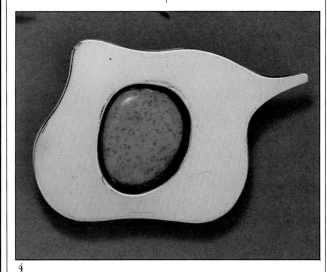

Artists have often turned their hand to jewelry design. Jean Arp (born 1888 in France) produced this rather surreal silver and pebble brooch in the 1950s (4). Salvador

Dali's imagery also translated particularly well into extravagant jewelry, and George Braque designed an impressive range in his later years.

4

Modernism affected designers all over Europe, but Scandinavia led the field with their profound modernist jewelry designs after the war. The firm of Georg Jensen, in Denmark, influenced many other jewelers with its progressive artistic policy. Its many different designers, were each credited by name for the individual pieces they contributed to Jensen's. The starkly simple gold pendant from the late 1950s or early 1960s) (3) is by Bent Gabrielson Pederson, and is typical of the Scandinavian style. The shift from decorative work blurred the dividing line between sculpture and jewelry. In the 1950s, the Pomodoro Brothers, in Italy, begun working and exhibiting as both sculptors and jewelers (5). Arnaldo (born 1926) studied architecture, sculpture, and stage design, Giorgio (born 1930) studied painting, graphic art, and sculpture.

5

ABSTRACT INNOVATORS

Until the Second World War everyone looked to France for the latest trends, from fashion to fine art. From the 1940s, America began to dominate the world with modern art and popular culture. Neither American styling, the cool, refined Scandinavian jewelry, nor the sculpturally formed work from Germany and Italy had many parallels in France. The concise elegance of this French gold torque from the 1950s (**1**) is atypical of the national trend. The rough surface texture of the cast rectangles and the spare curve of wire owe their origins to Scandinavia, but the overall delicacy produced by the softness of the chain gives it a French flavor.

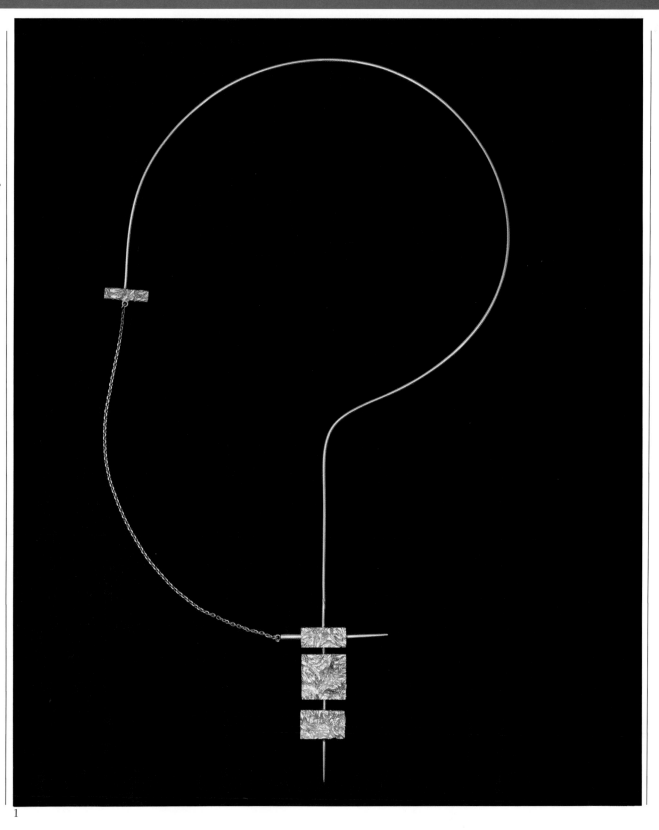

1

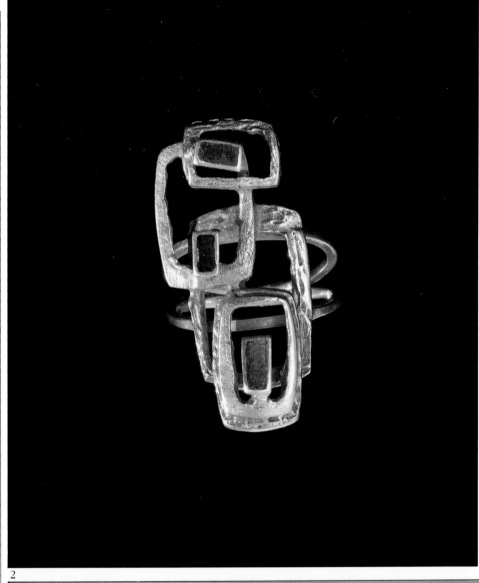

Abstraction in painting was the
most significant development this
century. The distillation of the
visual imagery filtered down to
every design discipline. This gold
and enamel ring (**2**) from the
1950s epitomizes the stylistic use of
rough rectangular forms, cast
metal with roughly textured
surface finishes, and powerful
colors used sparingly for
maximum effect. The gold,
diamond, and emerald bracelet
(**3**) by John Donald (born 1938),
shows how the new breed of art
college-trained jewelers embraced
modernism and experimentation
with individual flair in the late
1950s and 60s. Donald was one of
the first to use natural crystals in
his work.

2

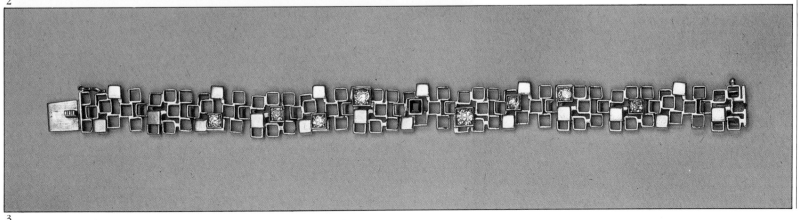

3

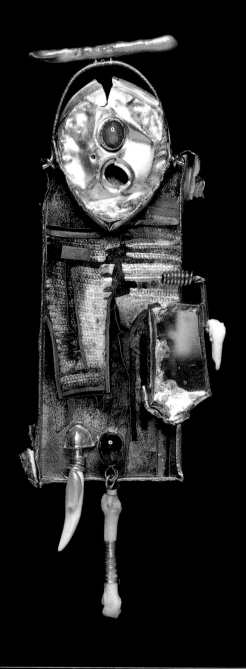

William Harper's "Temptation of Anthony," in gold cloisonné enamel on silver, gold, aluminum, opal, tourmaline, mirror, freshwater pearl, ivory, and bone.

CHAPTER NINE

CONTEMPORARY JEWELERS

1960-1989

Abstraction

·

Modern materials

·

Jewelry as art

·

Imagery from space and technology

HELEN CRAVEN

INTRODUCTION

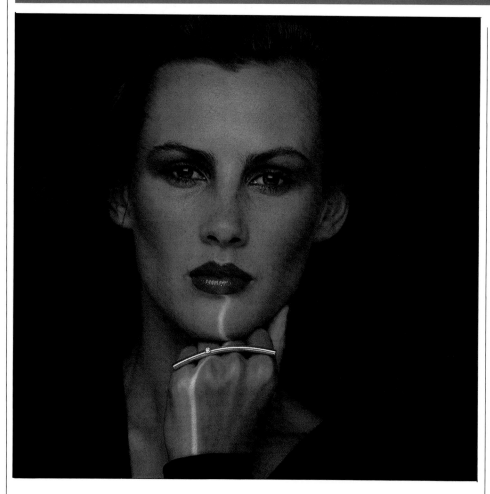

The stark simplicity of minimalism achieves a different perspective when applied to jewelry. Friedrich Becker uses simple forms, as in this gold and diamond ring, but his concern is to make his pieces come to life with the natural movements of the wearer. The curves of the body and the curves created by movement transform his technical forms into inspired expressiveness.

In the last 30 years, the Western world has experienced unprecedented technological advances, with immense social changes following in their wake. Although jewelry – as a decorative art – has never been in the vanguard of cultural change, many contemporary jewelers have reflected changing social mores by using their ingenuity and expertise to explore the medium and even question its values.

Continuing Traditions

Not all has been change, though. The most famous names in the jewelry world – Cartier, Bulgari, Boucheron, Asprey and Tiffany – have remained faithful to their exclusive and wealthy clientele and continue to produce jewelry in the traditional "grand manner." The established companies still devise sumptuous designs in precious metals and exquisite gemstones as status symbols, heirlooms and investments. In recent years many consumers of this grand jewelry have been from the Middle East, where tradition still demands the formal display of wealth and rank.

In England, the 1960s brought a new generation of artist-jewelers, as well as a new wealthy, self-made clientele. There was a great demand for a different species of jewelry: less formal, more modern, and an expression of the affluent decade.

In 1961 the Worshipful Company of Goldsmiths held an influential milestone exhibition of modern jewelry which revealed the potential of jewelry as a medium for artistic self-expression. 1960s British jewelry, epitomized by the work of Andrew Grima, was self-consciously modern, aiming to break with the past. Grima, for example, came to jewelry making from engineering. In 1946, he began producing traditional jewelry for his own H.J. company, although by 1961 he was taking a much freer approach. Many of his works were based on *objets trouvés*. He managed to capture the texture of leaves, twigs, and bark in precious metal, casting his pieces in 18-carat gold and studding them with gemstones.

Alongside Grima, jewelers such as John Donald, Louis Osman, Gillian Packard, and David Thomas also developed contemporary designs using new images celebrating scientific achievement – for example molecular and cell structures. Materials were chosen more for their aesthetic value than for their monetary worth. Natural organic shapes were incorporated in the designs; uncut crystals and minerals were often used.

Gradually semiprecious stones such as tiger's eye, coral, lapis lazuli, and black onyx took over from crystals. Nonprecious stones were popular, and when precious stones were used they were an integral part of an overall design, not clustered together for their own sake.

In New York Jean Schlumberger reigned supreme over Tiffany in the 1960s, and he too was responsible for shifting the emphasis away from valuable stones and toward "artistic" content in design. Schlumberger had progressed from making costume jewels for Schiaparelli in Paris in the 1930s to making real, exotic, fantasy jewels in New York in the 1940s and 50s. In 1956 Walter Hoving invited Schlumberger to set up his own department in Tiffany, and to become vice-president of the store. Schlumberger embarked on a series of fantastic, rich, and sumptuous jewels, tinged with baroque splendor, created through the 50s, 60s and 70s. Schlumberger's subject matter was almost always organic, sometimes heraldic, always luscious and startling, reflecting the curiosities and marvels of nature. He loved color and dared to mix sapphires and emeralds, amethysts and aquamarines, spinels, turquoises, with lavish quantities of warm yellow gold and brilliant enamels.

In the 1960s, the artistic approach was taken much further. Theories of the Bauhaus continued to influence many art education institutions and designers throughout Europe. They encouraged the search for a universal, rational, simple beauty – a "democracy" of form. This influence can been seen throughout Europe well into the 1970s, particularly in Holland and Britain, and although there have been many other theories and methods of teaching design since, the rigors of the Bauhaus teaching, with its desire to define forms in a minimal way, are still held as fundamentals by many designers.

Jewelry as Art

The art world in the 1940s and 50s was dominated by the American Abstract Expressionists. Artists saw themselves as pioneers, liberating the world from the bonds of tradition. These ideas pervaded the whole world of art and design, and found expression in what were called Studio Crafts which usually demanded that a single individual be responsible for both designing and making unique hand-crafted pieces. In the US itself, Australia, Britain and many other countries, the teaching of Studio Crafts became a part of the art school curriculum, and jewelry making found a new role as an expressive art form.

Meanwhile, in Germany and France, the apprenticeship system remained strong, and the skill of the jeweler was respected as such. German art colleges still teach rigorous technical courses as well as fine art, and many teachers are noted jewelers in their own right: Herman Jünger, at the Munich Academie der bildenden künste; Friedrich Becker, in Düsseldorf; and Reinhold Reiling, in Pforzheim, for example. Reiling trained as an engraver as well as a goldsmith, and his early pieces were geometric and strongly influenced by Scandinavian designers. By the late 1960s, his work had become free and asymmetric. He studded his pieces with cabochon and facet-cut stones and began introducing texture. There is also a freedom from traditional restraint that characterizes American work, and the influence of the North and South American Indians is detectable. Their bold expressiveness can be seen in the work of many jewelers, such as Robert Ebendorf, William Harper, Mary Lee Hu, Richard Mawdsley, Stanley Lechtzin, Earl Pardon and many more. Many of America's leading jewelers are also teachers passing on their experience and enthusiasm to new generations of artist–jewelers.

With the breaking down of traditional barriers between different art disciplines, an increasing number of jewelers have presented their work as art. In England, David Watkins, of the Royal College of Art in London, first trained as a sculptor and then turned to jewelry. His neckpieces and bracelets have always appeared like sculptures that fit on and relate to the human body, rather than as anything purely decorative. His work has usually been exhibited in galleries with an artist's eye and attitude guiding its considered presentation. Dr Kevin Coates is very much an artist who has chosen to express his ideas and themes through sculptural jewelry design, using precious and semiprecious materials. Both spiritual and intellectual, the

brilliant jewels or miniature sculptures all tell a story, perpetuate a timeless myth, or bring a creature to life. David Courts and Bill Hackett work mainly to commission in precious materials. Their designs are characterized by a sleek sensuality, their themes taken from unusual, often macabre, aspects of nature: a frog's skeleton, for example, or a crayfish.

This growing more toward "artistic" could be seen developing among several other jewelers in the early 1970s. Certain German jewelers, noted for their technical excellence and attention to detail, also presented their designs as "pictures." Ulrike Bahrs and Norbert Muerrle produced figurative, pictorial pieces in forms that served either as jewelry or as graphic images. Gerd Rothman presented stickpins in a frame with a painted background. Gijs Bakker and Robert Smit, from Holland and Claus Bury, from Germany showed an affinity with Conceptual Art in

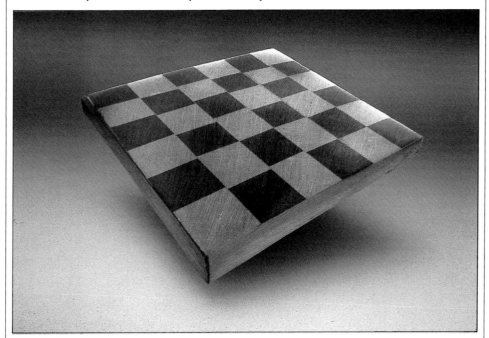

being concerned as much with showing their ideas as with exhibiting a finished product. Helga Zahn, from Britain showed Art Language to be her influence, with a 1975 brooch that included the words: "The philosophers have only inter preted the world in various ways, the point however is to change it. Marx."

New Concepts, New Materials, New Techniques

Inevitably, when jewelers were placed alongside fine artists and other designers, they were caught up in the desire of the younger generation for a voice and identity of its own. In the boom years of the 1960s, reflecting the sexual revolution that was taking place in the West, there

Many jewelers in the last twenty years have experimented with combinations of different metals for contrasts in color, texture, and form. Traditionalists have frowned on combining precious and base metals, but the ends often justify the means, as can be seen in this brooch by Barbara Christie made of silver and nickel.

INTRODUCTION

were significant changes in the fashions designed and worn by young people. Younger designers responded also to the social changes that were spreading across Europe.

In Britain, a "non-conformist" jeweler who stands out at this time is Gerda Flockinger. In 1961, when she was appointed to run the new jewelry course at Hornsey College of Art, she developed a program that not only taught traditional skills, but also encouraged experimentation. Her own work exhibited an irreverence to the traditional treatment of precious metals. She melted the surfaces of her jewelry to exploit the natural texture that was created by a combination of skill and accident. She fused wire and shapes cut from sheet metal, setting semi-precious stones and pearls into the finished form so that they appeared like intriguing decorative blisters, bubbling from the surface. The overall impression is of an organic form that has grown miraculously rather than of a fabricated artefact.

Patricia Tormey went even further, slamming molten gold between layers of textured charcoal or dropping it into a tray of lentils. Her best-known pieces, though, are minute, often erotic, tableaus cast in gold.

In Holland, traditionally trained jewelers Gijs Bakker and Emmy van Leersum turned the very notion of jewelry on its head when they experimented with the simple forms that became both clothing and jewelry. They also made large neckpieces that imposed physical constraints on the wearer. Their questioning of the nature of jewelry affected many other jewelers in Europe, particularly in Britain and their native Holland. When did jewelry become clothing? When did it become unwearable? When did it become sculpture? These questions continued to be asked for the next 15 to 20 years.

Some contemporary jewelers have shown an awareness of particular political issues, and their work has included social comment as well as visual statements about their chosen medium. David Poston, for example, protested against the poor working conditions and exploitation of the black miners in South Africa by exhibiting in 1975 a forged-steel neckpiece, shaped like a manacle and with the words "Diamonds, gold and slavery are forever" inlaid in

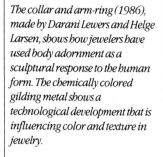

The collar and arm-ring (1986), made by Darani Lewers and Helge Larsen, shows how jewelers have used body adornment as a sculptural response to the human form. The chemically colored gilding metal shows a technological development that is influencing color and texture in jewelry.

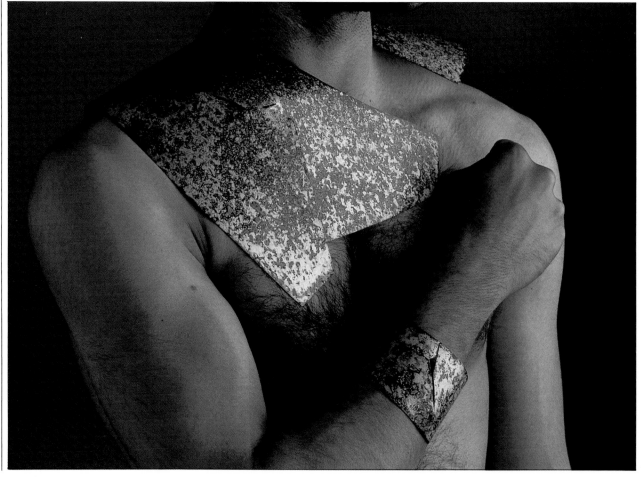

silver. Some simply rejected the use of precious metals and gemstones because of their high cost and the elitism they represented.

Australia is now beginning to establish a jewelry style of its own. During the 1960s and 70s many European jewelers visited, conducting workshops and exhibiting their work there. Initially this led to a spate of derivative work from the newly graduating students which fed an existing trade invariably run by immigrants from Europe. However, the seeds had been sown and students began to experiment with jewelry as a means of self expression. Soon jewelers emerged with a distinctive Australian feel. Wolf Wennrich, Helge Larsen, and Darani Lewers have been the key figures in this development, while Frank Bauer, who trained in Germany, Anne Brownsworth, Susan Cohn, Rowena Gough, Peter Tully, and Lyn Tune are just a few of the new generation of Australian jewelers producing increasingly interesting results.

In the 1970s imagery from space hardware and micro-technology was captured in jewelry form by Pierre Degen (a Swiss now working in Britain), the Australian Fritz Maierhofer and the Englishman Roger Morris. They used metal and colored plastics in combination, with finishes that were reminiscent of machine-made products. The forms sometimes seemed more concerned with the sculptural than the wearable and had enough presence to stand alone. Roger Morris even made sculptural pieces that included jewelry within them that could then be taken out and worn.

In Holland, Bakker, and Leersum rejected precious metals and used metals previously associated with industrial manufacture instead. Their idea was to show that even if a metal is neither rare nor expensive it can have aesthetic qualities. They were also continuing the Bauhaus tradition of gearing their designs for mass-production.

The idealistic notion that "good" and "innovative" design could be made available to all was taken up by various jewelers. However, manufacturers have remained steadfastly resistant to taking risks, so this has remained an ideal rather than a reality. Innovative jewelers also create their own elitism, however unwittingly, through a preciousness in style rather than materials. Despite this, there is little doubt that the innovators have influenced the more commercial end of costume jewelry – which makes the originals the more collectable.

The use of different materials, from platinum to paper, has brought infinite variety into the world of jewelry. And space technology has contributed materials, as well as imagery, to jewelry design – particularly the refractory metals ranging from niobium, which is the same density as gold, to titanium, which is very light and strong. But their most interesting property is that they are capable of changing their surface until they reflect every color of the spectrum. Edward de Large, now working in the US, was one of

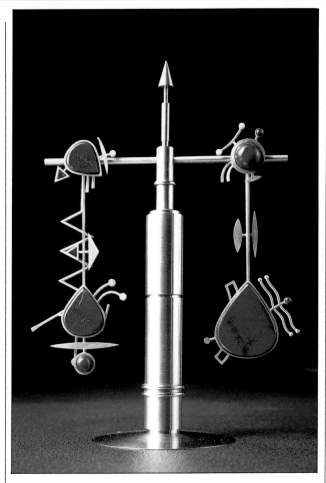

the first to perfect the use of refractory metals for jewelry, creating beautiful illusionistic landscapes on brooches and pendants.

The Style and Post-Modernism

Today's jewelers are again reflecting cultural trends, using the pluralism associated with Post-Modern culture to widen their scope. The political aspects of jewelry have diminished. Decoration without an added meaning is acceptable again.

A greater element of fun has also crept into body adornment. The Englishman Geoff Roberts, formerly a student of sculpture and printmaking, works with plastic and brightly colored metal foil to produce deliberately cheap jewelry that is essentially a combination of fun and fantasy. The Swiss Otto Kunzli, who studied under Hermann Jünger in Munich, uses a more satirical wit with such things as large three-dimensional brooches covered in "tasteless" wallpaper. And fine artist Peter Chang has hit the headlines with his large, brightly colored bangles in vacuum-formed plastic. Only time will tell how they will endure.

Sculptural objects that become jewelry or jewelry that becomes sculpture are results of the jewelry revolution of the 1960s and 70s. Wendy Ramshaw is notable for her sculptural stands which display her ring sets. She began making stands for her jewelry in the 1970s, and this earring stand from 1988 shows that her ideas and forms continue to develop and intrigue the viewer.

INFLUENCES

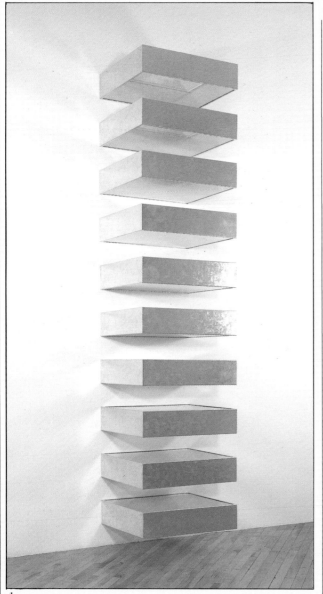

1

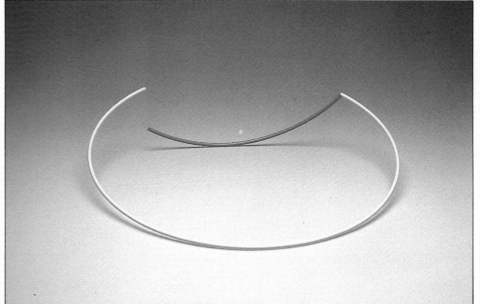

2

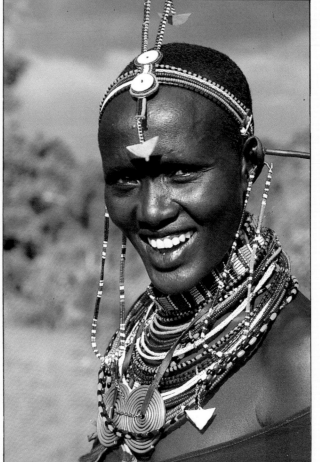

3

A fascinating correlation can be seen between the work of jewelers like Lam de Wolf, from Holland (**4**), and traditional tribal jewelry (**3**). Jewelers who create total body adornments seem to be expressing a basic human need for ritual and symbolic ceremony that is nowadays lacking in our lives. The beautiful Masai woman wears jewelry that is exciting and joyful, a real celebration of life and beauty, but it is also very complex. It must have taken many careful hours, not only to make, but also to put on.

Movements in fine art inevitably affect experimental jewelers, and the Minimalist sculptors who emerged in the 1970s had their counterparts among jewelers, particularly in Holland. Forms were refined and simplified to the extreme, occasionally using repetition to add power and emphasis, as with the galvanized iron and clear Plexiglas sculpture (**1**) by Donald Judd from 1985. Dutch jeweler Herman Hermsen has reduced his neckpiece (**2**) to one clear dynamic line, but with subtle changes of curve to give it a three-dimensional quality.

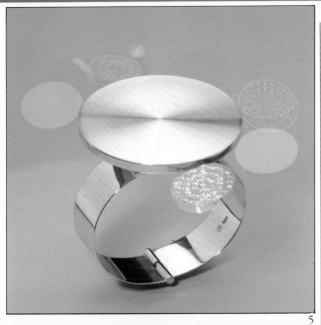

One of the themes of youth culture of the early 1960s was the future seen as some kind of science-fiction adventure. Space-age clothing, pioneered by Courrèges, materialized from Paris. The "Cosmos" dress from Balmain (**6**) in 1967 exhibited the trend toward simple geometric shapes and shorter hemlines. Friedrich Becker's kinetic jewelry illustrated the same geometric dynamism. He started introducing parts moved in response to the wearer in 1965. The white-gold and diamond bangle (**5**) dates from 1970.

5

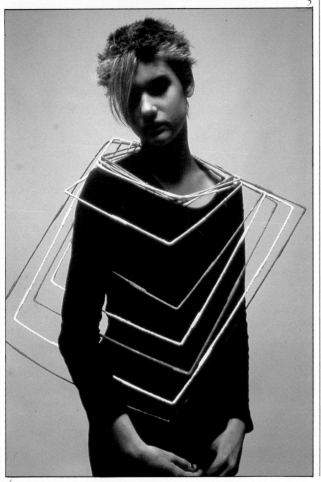

4

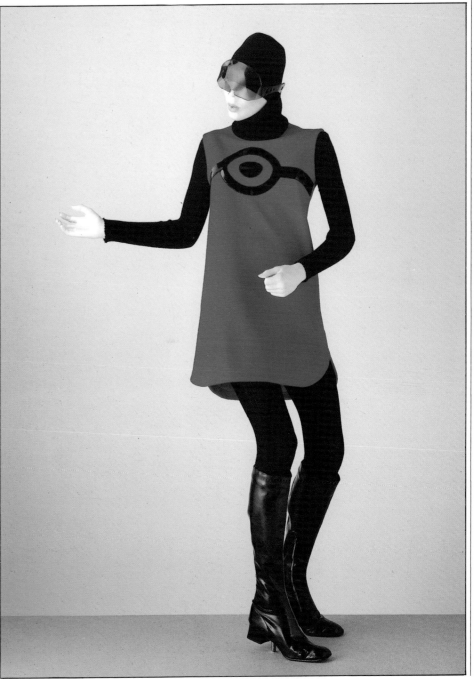

6

MAINSTREAM MODERN

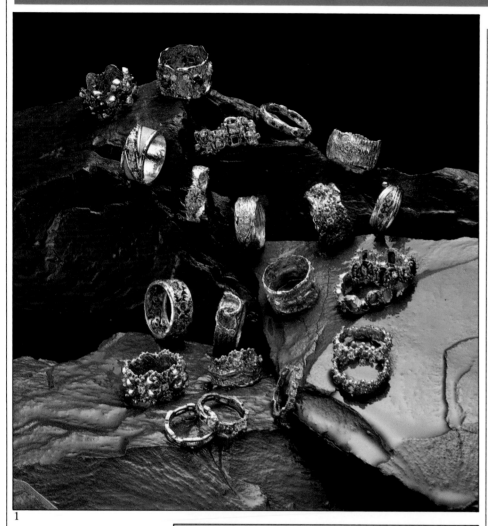

1

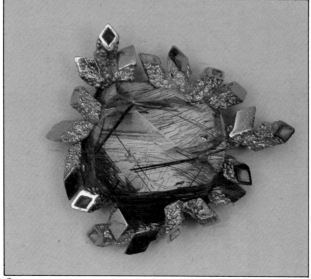

2

Andrew Grima (born 1921) has developed his own original approach to designing jewelry (**3**). Although he has adopted the contemporary trend for texture, abstract shapes, and even the use of objets trouvés, he creates an extravagant and opulent end product. The British royal family have bought his jewels both for themselves and for State gifts.

David Thomas (born 1938) set up his own workshop in the 1960s after studying at the Royal College of Art in London. Working instinctively, he liked to build up his pieces organically rather than by designing in detail on paper first. He made pieces like the swirling gold wire and diamond brooch (**4**) piece by piece, soldering with a micro-welder.

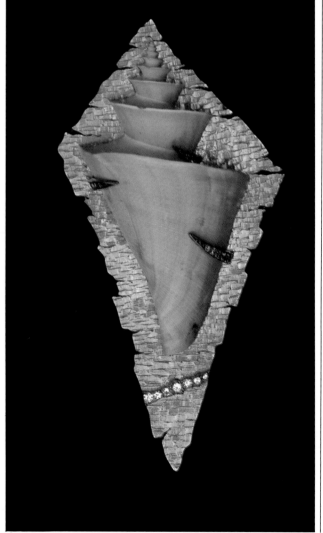

3

New jewelers in the 1960s designed for the mainstream gold and diamond market, but developed innovative ideas. Charles de Temple came from an unusual background; although he now lives in London, his father was Tom Mix, the famous American cowboy. His jewelry was equally unconventional. His wedding rings (**1**) exemplify his encrusted and heavily textured finishes. John Donald's brooch with rutilated quartz (**2**) shows his inventive use of gold in a surround that seems to continue in a natural crystalline form from the stone.

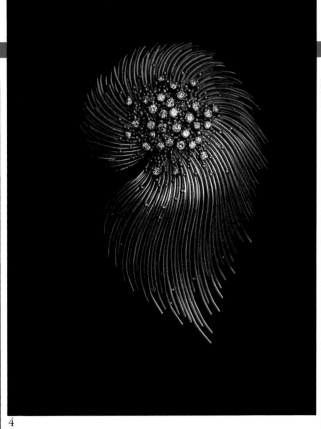

4

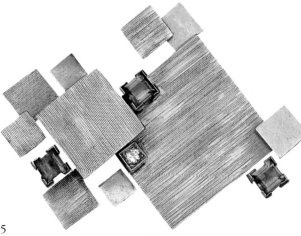

5

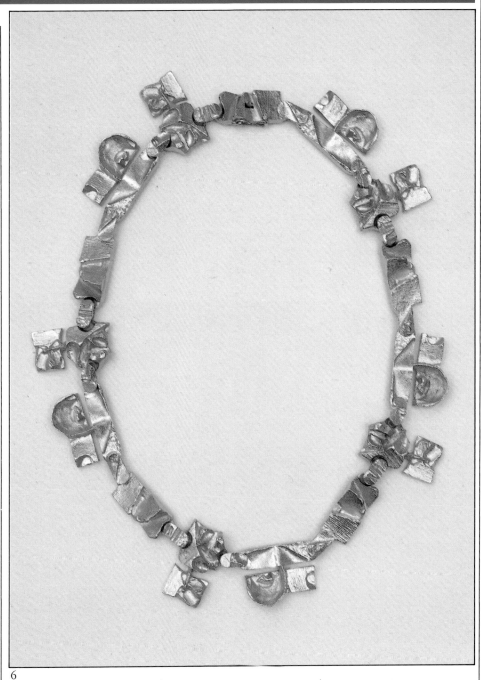

6

The geometry of the 1960s is noticeably more hard-edged than that of Art Deco designs. The brooch (**5**) by Gillian Packard, in different colored golds with emeralds and diamonds, has more to do with the bas relief pictures of someone like Ben Nicholson than with traditional jewelry ornamentation. Gillian Packard, born in 1938, was a graduate of the Royal College of Art in London. She is better known for her rings, which were often sensually curving and easy to wear. Her ingenious wedding and engagement ring sets would neatly slot together, a style that many were to emulate.

Björn Weckström's impressive necklace (**6**) uses gold with supreme confidence. The bold, nuggety segments have no need of gemstones. Weckström was born in Helsinki in 1935 and worked for the famous Lapponia Jewelry company there. He now has his own gallery, also in Helsinki, and belongs to the Finnish Sculptors' Union as well as ORNAMO, the designers' union. There is an increasing acceptance that jewelers can be sculptors and vice-versa, although resistance from the more traditional art academies is vehement.

NON-CONFORMISM

GERDA FLOCKINGER

The most influential jeweler working in Britain in the 1950s was Gerda Flockinger. Although there were changing attitudes in America and other parts of Europe, whereby jewelers presented their work as art, Britain demonstrated a more traditional approach, and few jewelers were prepared to step outside the bounds of acceptability. Flockinger inspired many of the new generation of experimental jewelers, not just with her technical approach, but with her attitude toward jewelry design and making. Born in 1927 in Innsbruck, she studied fine art at St Martin's School of Art in London from 1945 to 1950. She then went on to study at the Central School of Art and Design from 1950 to 1955, where she took up jewelry as well as etching and enameling. She was one of the first jewelers to be given a one-person exhibition at the Arnolfini Gallery in Bristol, which signified an important step in jewelry

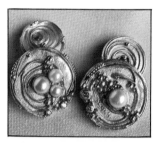

1983 cufflinks in silver, 18-carat gold, diamonds and cultured pearls.

development. It was as a result of the work, attitudes, and personalities of jewelers like Gerda Flockinger that it became usual for jewelry to be seen in galleries and in exhibitions. When she inaugurated a jewelry course at Hornsey College of Art (now Middlesex Polytechnic) in London in 1962, she had a more direct influence on new jewelers. The course was exciting and experimental, and Middlesex is still considered an important and prestigious place to study. David Poston and Charlotte de Syllas both studied with her. David Poston used his work to express his political views in the early 1970s, while Charlotte de Syllas developed a profound independence from familiar trends. It is noticeable that they each found a unique means of self-expression, no doubt helped by their college environment.

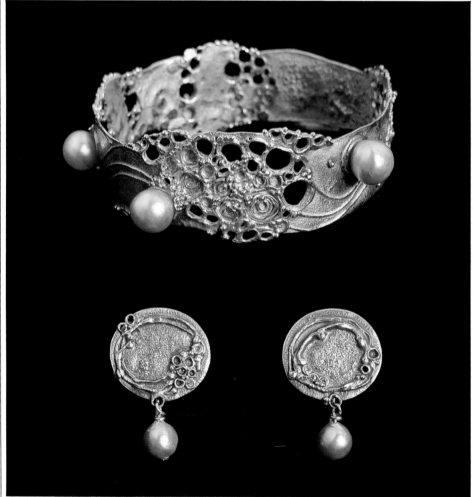

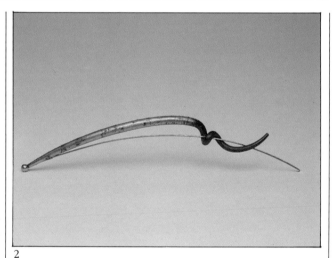

2

*The bangle and earrings (**1**) show Gerda Flockinger's individual style, with adeptly melted metal sheet and fused lines of wire. The bangle (1973) is made from silver and pearls, and the earrings (1975) are intricately constructed of silver with oxides and 18-carat gold. She has subtly included small brilliant-cut diamonds in the earrings, and finished them with hanging pearls.*

*Elisabeth Holder's technical excellence reflects her German training. Born in Sindelfingen, in West Germany, in 1950 she undertook an apprenticeship training as well as art college study. She came to London and studied again at the Royal College of Art, finally setting up her workshop in London in 1980. Her brooch (1988) shows a masterly use of metals, with a typically elegant and simple but expressive design that stretches out and ends with a flourish (**2**).*

1

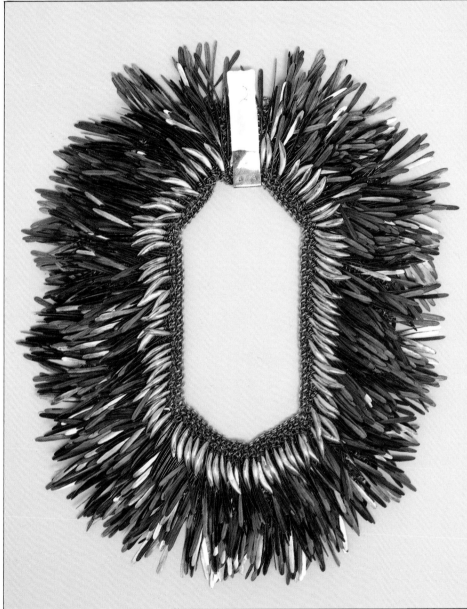

3

Many British jewelers in the 1970s abandoned precious metals in favor of other materials. Catherine Mannheim has stayed with metal, but not with tradition. She has used the imagery of Pop art – words spelled out in raised letters, figurative pictures, and sometimes photographs framed behind glass – for a brooch. Her amphorae brooch (4) is fused silver with applied gold (1986).

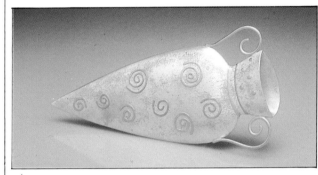

4

Jewelry in the past was often related to myth, magic, and ceremony; and the work of Tone Vigeland seems to echo the Nordic traditions of such symbolic and efficacious jewelry. She was born in Oslo in 1938 and studied at the Kunst & Handverksskolen there from 1955 and at Oslo Yrkesskole from 1957. She established her own workshop in 1961. The dramatic and feather-like necklace (3) is made from silver, steel, and gold with mother-of-pearl in the clasp (1983).

Hand-worked metal, made with the mind, the hand, and the heart can create the fetish objects of our urban age. The symbolism is timeless, and the jewelry is essentially precious and compelling. Cynthia Cousens's hatpins (5) in copper, gold, steel, and silver are very much more than the sum of their parts or merely the result of technical skill.

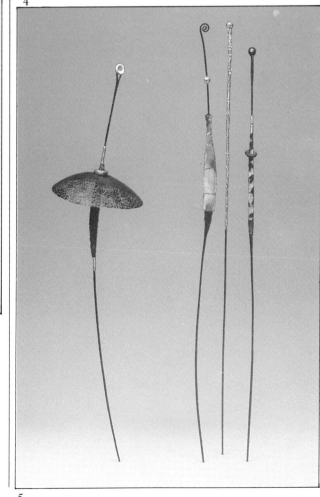

5

173

NON-CONFORMISM

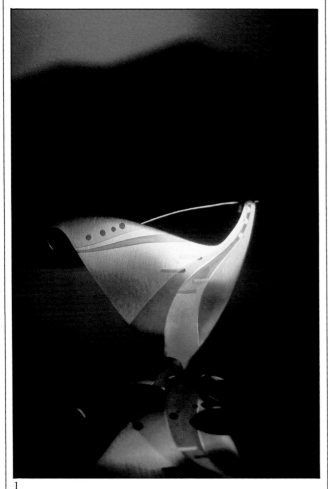

1

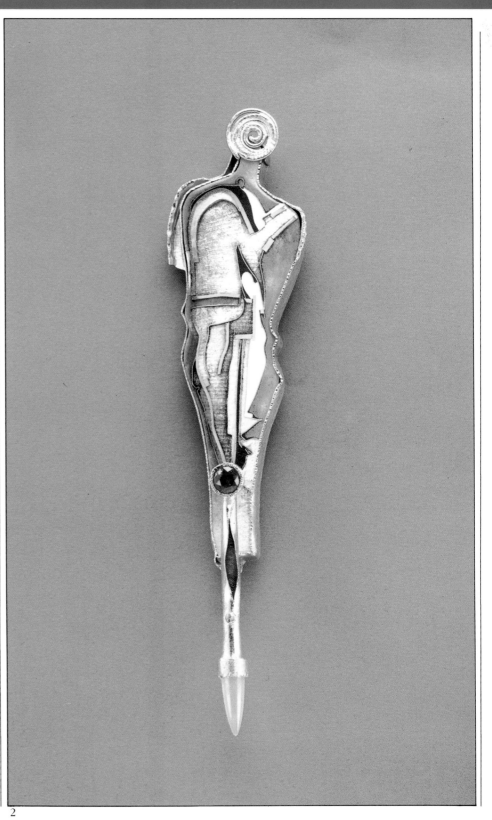

*Refractory metals provided a new resource for jewelers in the 20th century. Their potential for vivid colors has made them very popular. Anne Marie Shillitoe was one of the pioneers in their use in Britain. Unlike the majority of exponents she uses them with subtlety in elegant curving forms. The fibula (**1**) is in anodized titanium inlaid with tantalum and niobium, c.1980.*

*William Harper follows his American jewelry pioneers in seeing his work as art. "The White Hermaphrodite" (**2**) is a brooch relating to his theme of the search for beauty and truth through dichotomy. He posits the idea that the perfect human would be both male and female. To create life takes a male and female, and to make art one must also be both.*

2

Australian jewelry in the 19th century used images of local flora and fauna. Helge Larsen and Darani Lewers have reflected this celebration of their surroundings with their "Kookaburra" pendant (**3**). They have been pioneers of the modern jewelry movement in Australia since 1961. They feel that their jewelry is a form of body language through which they can express their ideas and feelings. When worn it can take on further meaning from the personality of the wearer.

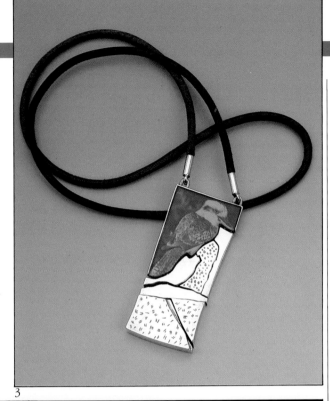

3

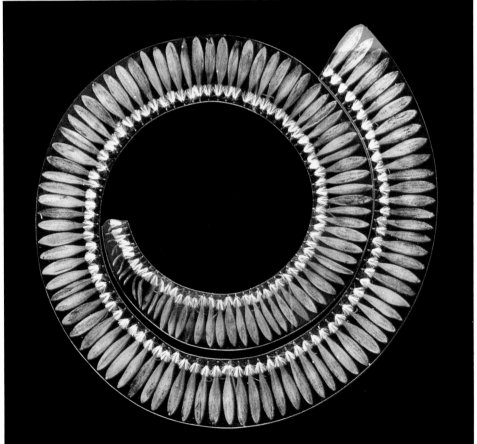

4

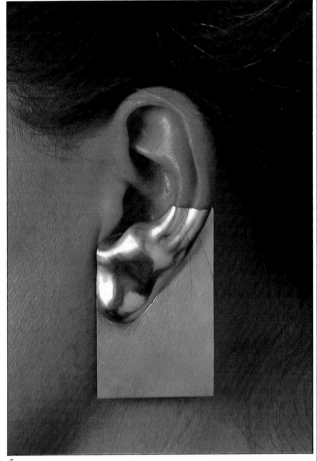

5

Sometimes the concept behind a piece of jewelry is more important than the finished piece. Gijs Bakker (born 1942 in Holland) has consistently managed to surprise even the most experimental. The necklace (**4**) of flower petals, which by nature are temporary and insubstantial, are preserved for posterity inside a carefully constructed spiral – man's attempts to control nature perhaps?

The highly personal nature of jewelry has been taken to an extreme by Gerd Rothman (born 1941 in Germany) who has cast small parts of individual people's bodies in silver. The earring (**5**) was made in 1984.

ABSTRACT AND NON-PRECIOUS PIECES

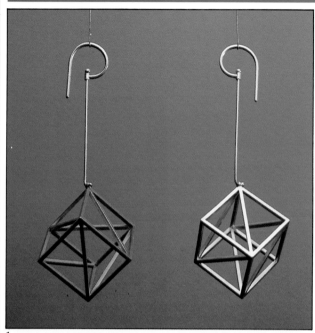

1

Fritz Maierhofer (born 1941 in Austria) is another jeweler noted for his precision pieces. He admits to being more concerned with structure and form than with wearability, although this does not mean they are not worn. In this recent girder-like pin (**3**), he has contrasted shiny yellow metal with oxidized white metal.

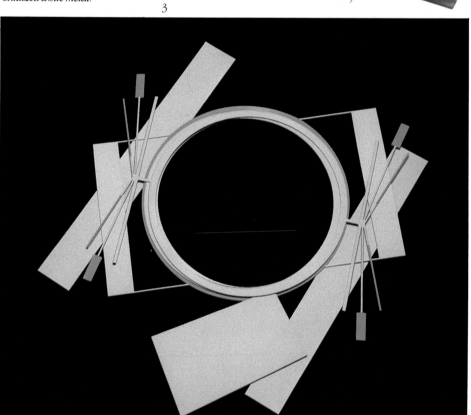

3

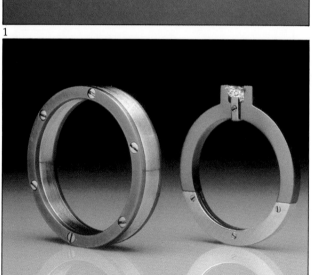

2

4

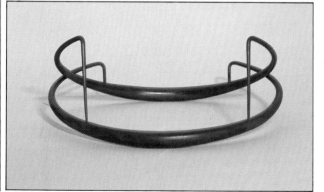

Frank Bauer (born in 1942 in Germany and now living in Australia) reveals his architectural background in his beautifully constructed geometric pieces. The cube earrings (**1**) are in 18-carat gold (1980). Joel Degen (born in 1941 in France, now living in London) shows his methods of construction in his 1980s wedding and engagement rings (**2**).

David Watkins (born 1940) is one of the leading contemporary jewelers in Britain. He has consistently produced impressive sculptural collections of jewelry, the later pieces being made from steel coated with colored neoprene. These necklaces can be worn separately or in combination (**4**).

David Poston (born 1948) has moved through various stages of development. He was one of the first jewellers to include textiles in his work, and caused a commotion when he made a huge necklace out of stones for an elephant! His later work has been very simple and refined like the neckpieces and bangles (1983) in steel and titanium (**5**).

5

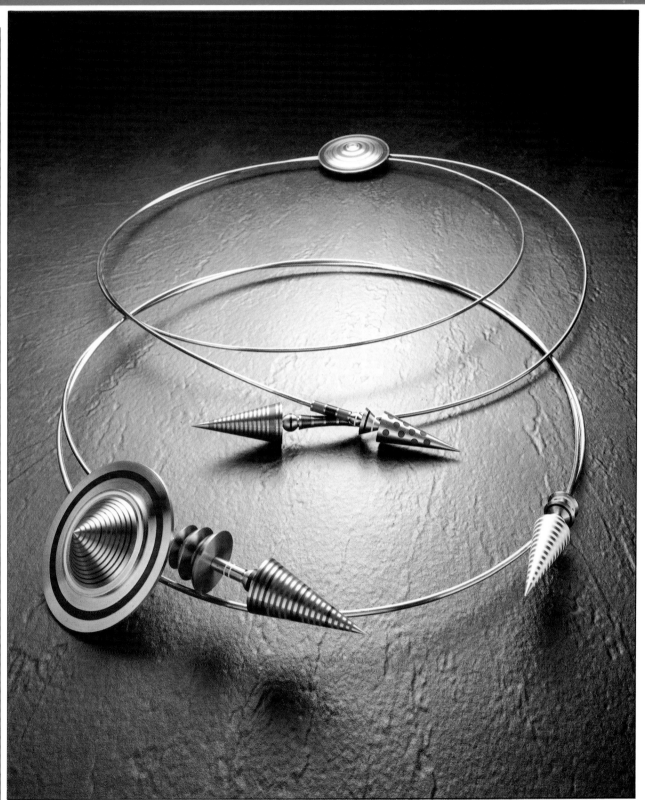

Wendy Ramshaw (born 1939) is one of the most successful contemporary jewelers to have emerged out of the 1970s. She has managed to combine fashion and innovation in her work, and her award-winning designs have proved to be extremely popular with the buying public. She first became known for her ring sets, which she presented on rocket-shaped stands. She turned the stands and parts of the rings on a lathe, but maintained a quality of feminine prettiness within her high-tech imagery. Although she has predominantly and skillfully used precious metals, she has also experimented with paper, glass, and porcelain, and even developed "performance art" pieces. The "Orbit" necklaces pictured here (6) were made in 1988.

6

COLOR AND FASHION

Fashion jewelers can often be freer and more spontaneous with their jewelry. The materials are cheaper and more easily marketed. Katzie Hughes screen-prints on paper and then embeds the paper in resin. With processes like these she can be more experimental with her shapes and colors (**2**).

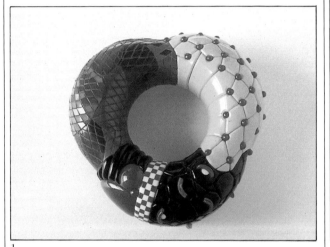

1

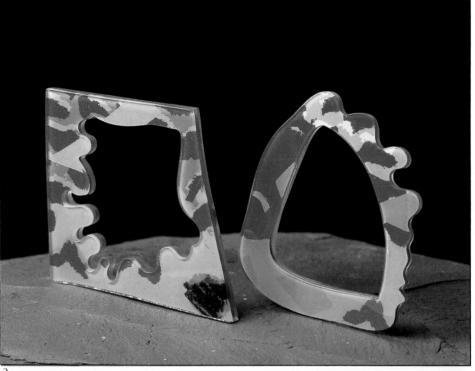

2

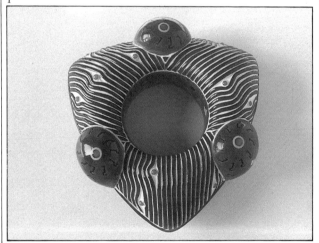

3

High-fashion jewelry is also now the province of the artist-jeweler. Peter Chang is primarily a fine artist, but his vacuum-formed plastic jewelry was recently used by Rifat Ozbeck for a fashion show. The bangles (**1** and **3**) are good examples of his dramatic and highly decorative creations.

Geoff Roberts is one of the most prolific and inventive fashion jewelers. He initially trained as a sculptor and then as a printmaker. His acrylic necklace (**4**) hints at the color, intensity, and preciousness of gems with the rich colors obtained from metal blocking foil.

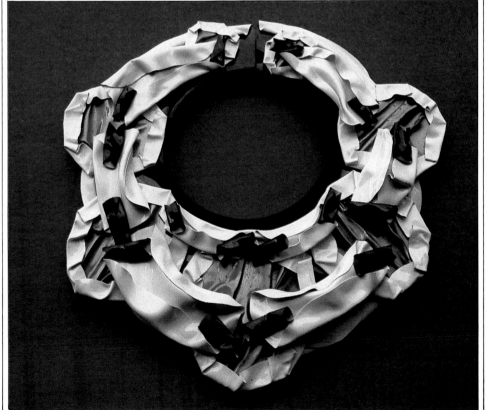

4

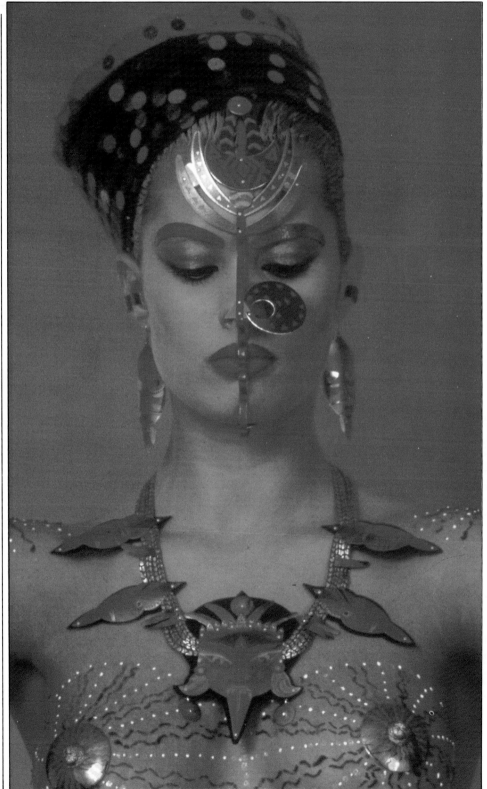

Titanium is a hard metal to fashion, but Clarissa (**5**) has managed to achieve great delicacy in her work. Her exotic imagery stems from her research in Indonesia, although her work has always involved complex color patterns and interesting shapes. During her studies at the Royal College of Art she experimented with coating different surfaces with an iridescent titanium color.

After the street style of Punk, it no longer seemed excessive to swathe oneself with paste jewels and strings of pearls. At a time when the British public was hungry for glamor, Monty Don brought out a range of large crystal and pearl drops topped with bows. Many more sumptuous designs followed. Current work includes large, glittering paste hanging baskets (**6**).

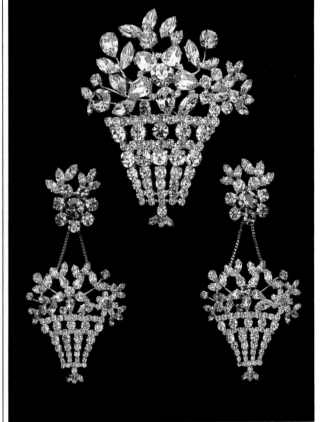

6

5

WEARABLE ART

Artist-jewelers sometimes include objects that relate to their jewelry alongside their wearable work largely by their scale and preciousness. Onno Boekhoudt (born 1944 in Holland) produced this group of objects (**1**) in 1984. He has proved to be an influential force in Dutch jewelry. He has shown a less clinical and altogether freer approach than that of his Minimalist contemporaries. He teaches at the Gerrit Rietveld Akademie, in Amsterdam, Holland's most prestigious design school.

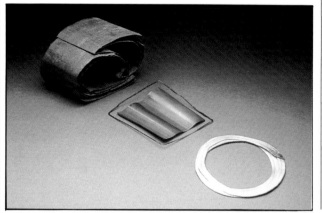

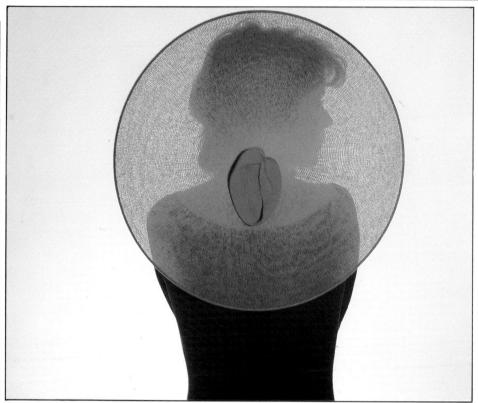

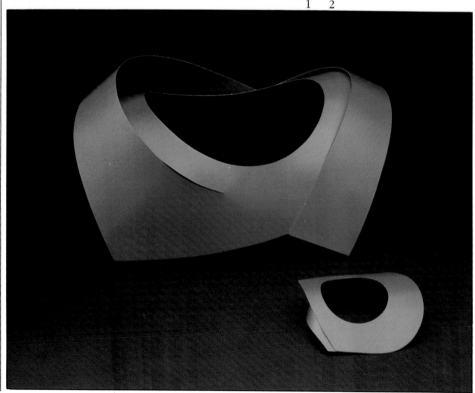

Susannah Heron (born 1949 in England) has proved to be one of the most thoughtful and inventive jewelers in Britain. As she moved toward more sculptural forms she called her work "Wearables" rather than jewelry. Her "Wearable: large turquoise and red hat," from 1982 (**2**), heralded her complete move from jewelry to sculpture.

Although some jewelry can stand on its own as sculpture, most sculptural pieces are still really completed only when they are placed on the human body. Helge Larsen and Darani Lewer's anodized aluminum collar and armring from 1986 (**3**) powerfully suggest the curves of the body and anticipate a wearer.

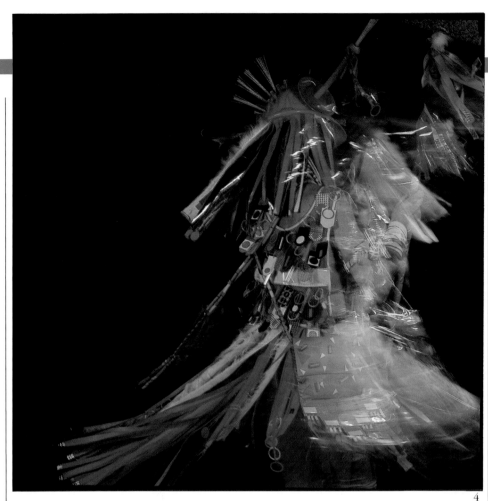

4

Peter Tully (born 1949) is an Australian who has developed an expressive, flamboyant and witty style which speaks volumes about his native country. A large exhibition of Australian jewelry which toured Europe in the early 1980s included his "Australian Belt," which consisted of brightly colored acrylic cutouts of Australian maps covered with cutout Vegemite labels, kangaroos, and Sydney Opera House. "Urban Tribalwear" (1981), is made from fluorescent vinyls, plastics, and rubber and comprises a headdress, breastplate, necklaces, bags, armbands, and skirt (4).

Gijs Bakker's is a more disturbing and calculated wit. His design techniques are cool and precise, but the end results can be startling. His idea of laminating photographs in clear plastic makes for a frighteningly realistic illusion (5). The necklace shown is entitled "Embracement" and dates from 1982.

When jewelry attempts to be witty it usually does so in a subtle and abstract way. But some jewelers exhibit their wit more overtly. Otto Kunzli (born in 1948 in Switzerland) studied metalwork in Zürich and jewelry in Munich under Hermann Jünger. His excellent training gives him all the more scope to subvert traditional jewelry values. His wit and ingenuity are matched by his craft and design skills. His dislike of jewelry as a status symbol or investment is epitomized in his replica of a gold bar made from cardboard (6).

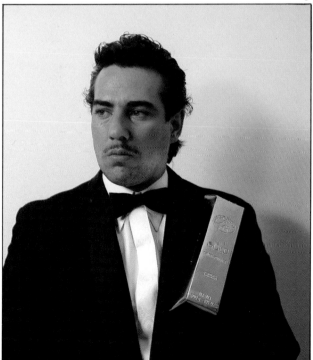

6

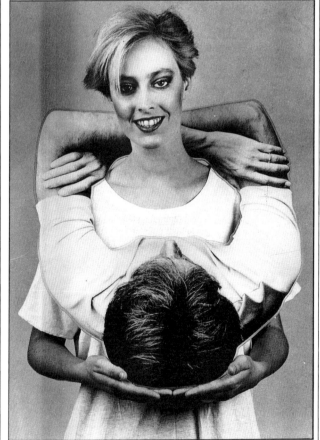

5

FIGURATIVE WORK

Figurative jewelry will never lose its appeal. Forms that are easily recognized can stir the emotions in an immediate and direct way. Charlotte de Syllas has never followed a particular trend with her jewelry and often works for many months on one piece so that when it finally leaves her hands it is exquisitely crafted and quite unique. The "Magpie" necklace (**1**) is made from black nephrite and white jadeite. The secondary feathers and tail are labradorite laminated onto black nephrite. The kumihino silk braids are by Catherine Martin.

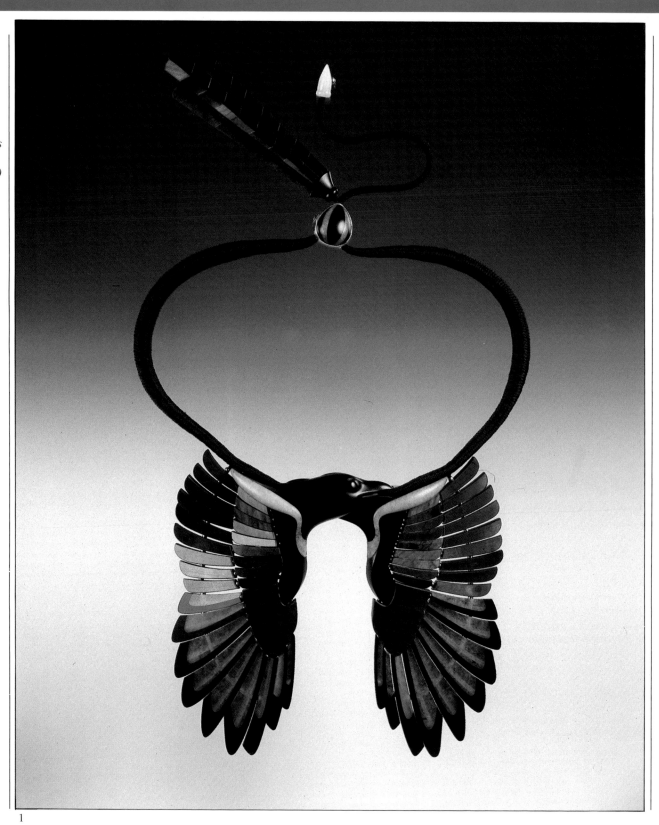

1

American jewelers are often uninhibited by design "traditions" and produce work that is idosyncratic and expressive of its maker's personality. Richard Mawdsley's narrative belt buckle (*2*), in sterling silver, lapis lazuli, and coral (1976), is entitled "Goneril, Regan, Cordelia." It combines the look of instrument parts and an expressionistic female form almost in the traditions of assemblage art. His virtuosity is particularly evident in his "Feast" bracelet (1974), which is a perfect miniature of a table set with jugs, goblets, dishes of food, wine buckets, and cutlery.

Sophie Chell shows a cooler, more British-influenced approach with her half jacket (*3*). Taking male stereotypes, she reduces them to brooch form with clever craft skills. Her brooches from 1980 utilize silver, silver-gilt, and niobium, materials with qualities that can be manipulated to represent particular images rather than to celebrate the materials themselves.

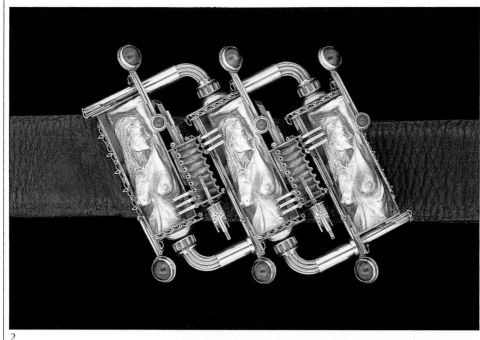

2

Bruno Martinazzi (born 1923 in Italy) is another artist who combines sculpture and jewelry. He originally studied chemistry and then psychology, before attending the State School of Art in Florence. His "Goldfinger" bracelet (*4*) dates from 1969. Viliama Grakalic (who was born in 1942 in Yugoslavia and moved to Australia in 1963) constantly uses the human form in her jewelry.

Her "Falling Man" brooch (*5*) is from a series of three.

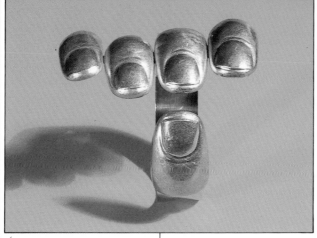

4

3

5

TOWARD THE FUTURE

Robert Ebendorf's feelings toward his jewelry are characteristic of many other artist-jewelers working in the 1980s. He wants to spark energy with his visual effects. He wants to encompass in his jewelry aspects of the life and culture that surround him; the experiences that we are all responding to in different ways. He wants to use his learned craft skills as a means to an end – to explore his creative potential – and make his finished work an expressive means of communication.

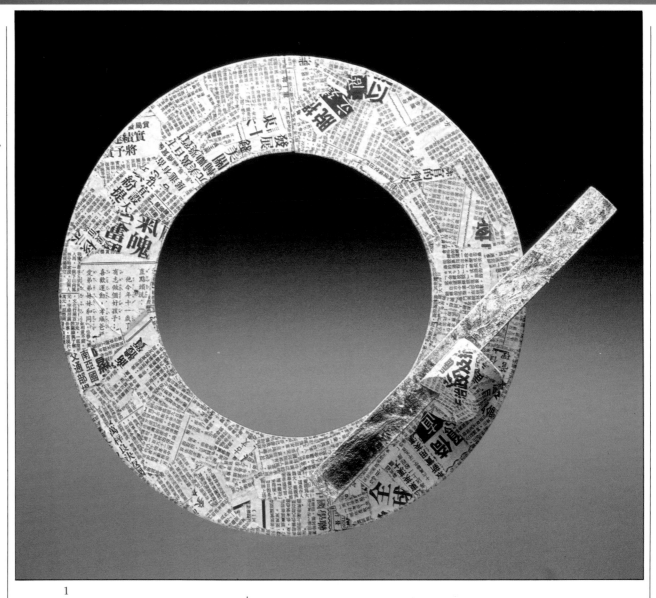

1

Two of his recent pieces are shown here. The neck-ring (*1*) measures 10 in (25 cm) in diameter and is constructed of an old Chinese newspaper and 24-carat gold foil. The mixed media necklace (*2*) is the same diameter; the heads are 2 in (5 cm) across.

Born in Kansas, in 1938, he received his master's degree in the fine arts. He has spent time in Norway studying and working at Norway Silver Design. He is currently Professor of Art at the State University of New York. Ebendorf is also a founding member and past President of the Society of North American

Goldsmiths, and in 1982 was honored as a Distinguished Member of the Society.

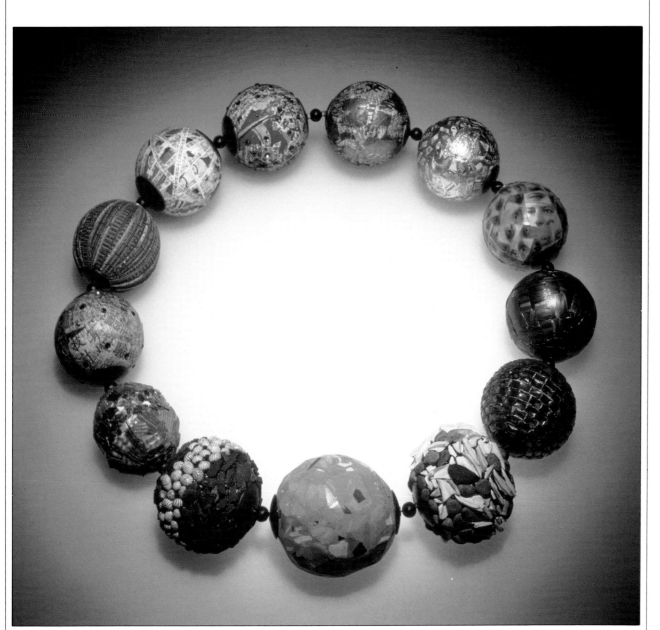

2

GLOSSARY

Acanthus: ornament based on the leaves of the Mediterranean Acanthus plant. Originally used to decorate the capitals of Corinthian columns.

Acrylic: a plastic resin used by some contemporary jewelers since the 1960s. It can be molded and cut, has a wide color range and is sometimes used in conjunction with metals.

Agate: a variety of CHALCEDONY, usually banded, in various colored layers alternating with milky white. Also MOSS-AGATE: a translucent gray, with green, black, or red inclusions of various oxides.

Aigrette (Fr.): a vertical hair ornament, usually jeweled, in the form of a plume of feathers or a spray of flowers.

Alexandrite: a type of CHRYSOBERYL, discovered in the Urals in 1831 and named after Tsar Alexander II. Occurs in red, white and green forms and is extremely light-sensitive, sometimes changing color from deep green to bright red.

Amazonstone (amazonite): a FELDSPAR varying from bright to bluish-green, it is opaque with an iridescent sheen. It cleaves easily, so is unsuitable for faceting and is usually cut EN CABOCHON.

Baguette (Fr.): a method of cutting gemstones in the shape of a long narrow rectangle bordered by four step-cut FACETS.

Bakelite: the trade name for the first thermosetting resin, patented in 1910 by Belgian doctor, Leo Baekeland. Used for the manufacture of early records, plastic wares, telephones, etc.

Balas ruby (also **spinel ruby**): misnomers for a spinel whose color resembles a ruby. The spinel is a bright transparent gemstone which occurs in many colors.

Baroque pearl: a large misshapen pearl, caused by an oyster pearl formation around an irregularly shaped inclusion.

Bas-relief: a relief, or projection from a surface, that is low or shallow.

Basse-taille (Fr.): an enameling technique in which translucent enamels are introduced over a ground which has been chased, engraved, or otherwise worked to create a modeled surface. The enamel color varies in intensity with the depth of the cutting.

Berlin Iron: originally early 19th-century cast-iron jewelry from the Berlin Iron Foundry. Most of it was produced in the period 1812-15, when pieces were presented in exchange for gold jewelry donated to the war-effort during the Napoleonic Wars. Some was also made in France.

Bezel: the principal component of a decorative finger ring, it surmounts the hoop encircling the finger. Term also used for the setting for a central stone or decoration.

Bijouterie (Fr.): a term that distinguishes jewelry made of gold and enamels from JOAILLERIE (Fr.), which is composed mainly of gemstones.

Biliment: a row of stones or pearls that bordered or transversed "gable" headdresses or French hoods in 16th-century England.

Blister pearl: an uneven, sometimes hollow pearl, with a raw underside which is usually hidden in a setting.

Bodkin: a long ornamental hairpin, of gold or silver set with gems; fashionable for fastening hair in the Renaissance.

Bracteate: a term used for a thin sheet of gold applied to pieces of jewelry, coins, medals etc.

Brilliant cut: a method of gem-cutting in which the upper part of the stone is cut in as many as 33 FACETS, and the lower part in 25. Particularly suited to diamonds.

Cabochon (Fr.): a stone with a smooth, curved, highly polished and unfaceted surface. The oldest method of gem-cutting still in use.

Caliber-cut (Fr.): a method of cutting usually small gemstones, to fit closely into groups or clusters which are massed around a main stone. Often an oblong or elliptical cut.

Cameo: a gem, hardstone or shell, of which the upper section is carved in relief while the lower serves as a ground.

Cannetille (Fr.): A particular type of FILIGREE used on jewelry settings, incorporating shells and burr-like motifs. Popular in France during the first half of the 19th century.

Carbuncle: almandine garnet cut en cabochon

Carcanet: bands of jewels worn as necklaces.

Carnelian: a translucent reddish CHALLEDONY; also spelled CORNELIAN

Cat's Eye: a general term for several varieties of gemstone which, in certain lights when cut en cabochon, exhibit a luminous moving line bisecting the stone. This is most notable in the lustrous yellowish-brown variety of CHRYSOBERYL.

Celluloid: the generic term for Pyroxylin (cellulose nitrate) plastics pioneered in Britain, but finally patented in the United States c. 1870 by the brothers James and Isaiah Hyatt.

Chalcedony: a variety of QUARTZ, usually of pale milky blue or gray, and evenly colored. It is porous so can be easily dyed to enhance or alter its color. Its several gemstone varieties include: AGATE, SARDONYX, CARNELIAN, CHRYSPOPRASE, ONYX.

Champlevé enamel (Fr.): an enameling technique in which individual compartments are created to receive the enamel by cutting away troughs or "cells" in the background metal. The enamel is then polished down to the level of the metal cells, forming a design.

Chaplet: a medieval hair ornament in the form of an encircling band of ornamental gold flowers and gemstones.

Chatelaine (Fr.): a decorative hook worn at the waist, from which are suspended on hooks or chains, various items for practical daily use in the household.

Chrysoberyl: said to derive from the Greek *chrysos* (gold) because of its typically golden-yellow color; it can vary to yellowish and bluish-green and brown. The most attractive and sought-after examples are the ALEXANDRTE and CAT'S EYE.

Chrysoprase: a variety of QUARTZ which occurs in shades of deep to yellowish-green and is usually cut en cabochon.

Citrine: the correct name for all yellow and pale brown varieties of QUARTZ and the most common yellow stone available.

Chrysoprase: a variety of QUARTZ which occurs in shades of deep to yellowish-green and is usually cut en cabochon.

Cloisonné enamel (Fr.): an enameling technique in which compartments or *cloisons* are built up from the metal background by attaching metal strips at right-angles to it. The *cloisons* are then filled in with enamel, their tops left exposed.

Collet: band of metal encircling a stone and holding it in place.

Collier de Chien (Fr.): or Dog Collar: a choker of many strands, usually of pearls or diamonds, sometimes with a central brooch or *plaque-de-cou*. A fashion popularized by Queen Alexandra, wife of Edward VII.

Coque de Perle (Fr.): a large, thin section cut from the central whorl of a shell of the Nautilus. It is irregularly shaped, very white and resembles somewhat the BLISTER PEARL.

Cornelian: a translucent reddish CHALCEDONY. Perhaps due to its fleshy color it is also known as CARNELIAN, from *carnis* (L. flesh).

Coronal: a simple open crown worn by Medieval noblemen and women, it is usually decorated with *fleurons*.

Cosse de Pois (Fr.): a decorative motif consisting of a repeated design of elongated leaf-shapes resembling pea-pods. Originated in France in the early 17th century.

Crocidolite: a fibrous mineral; its color ranges from mauve to green. When decomposed as quartz it can change to a golden brown, which is known as a TIGER'S EYE.

Email en ronde bosse (Fr.): a type of painted enameling in which the enamel is applied to figures or other modeling in high relief. Also known as encrusted enameling.

En plein (Fr.): a term describing the application of enamel directly to a surface rather than to plaques attached to it.

En tremblant (Fr.): a technique in which parts of large, ornamental, usually floral, jewels are set on tiny springs which quiver or "tremble" when worn.

Esclavage (Fr.): literally, slavery; a necklace comprising three chains or strings of jewels or beads which are equidistant.

Feldspar: the name for a large group of minerals. Though of geological importance, few are suitable for gemstones. These include MOONSTONE and AMAZONSTONE.

Ferronière (Fr.): a hair ornament in the form of a chain encircling the head, with a pendant which falls at the center of the forehead.

Filigree: delicate silver or gold wire threads designed in complex repeating patterns.

Foil: an ancient means of improving the color and brilliance of stones by backing them with a thin leaf of highly polished metal.

Fret: a geometrical ornament of intersecting horizontal and vertical lines repeated to form a pattern.

Garnet: a gemstone popular from antiquity, the name derives from *granatum* (L.) for pomegranate, a reference to its color. Its six varieties include: ALMANDINE: dark crimson in color and often cut en cabochon, when it is known as a CARBUNCLE;

DEMANTOID: green in color, its name refers to its diamond-like sparkle, it is often used as a series of tiny stones surrounding a larger gem; and HESSONITE: transparent yellow, orange or brownish in color. Also known as "cinnamon stone" and "jacinth."

Giardinetto (It.): literally, small garden: a type of late 17th to 18th century ring of openwork floral design, set with various colored gems.

Gimmel: derived from *gemellus* (L. a twin): the name for a ring that separates into two interlinked parts.

Girandole: a type of earring or brooch in which three pendant drops are suspended from a larger bow-shaped setting.

Granulation: An Etruscan gold-working technique, revived in the 19th century, in which minute grains of gold are applied to a metal surface forming patterns in low relief.

Greek cross: a cross with four equidistant arms of equal size.

Hardstone: a loose term generally applied to opaque semi- or non-precious stones.

Intaglio: the opposite of CAMEO; a method in which a design is carved into the surface of a gemstone or hardstone.

Jasper: closely related to AGATE, its many impurities cause its coloration of red, brown, yellow, or green. It is more common than CHALCEDONY and a popular stone for carving.

Jerusalem cross: a cross with four equidistant and equally sized arms which terminate in flanged ends.

Joaillerie (Fr.): see BIJOUTERIE

Lapis Lazuli: a complex mineral of an intense purply-blue, sometimes with inclusions of sparkling pyrites. Widely used for decoration and ornament. Because of its colour and resistance to fading, it was also ground for use as a pigment for the paint colour Ultramarine. The name possibly originated in the Middle Ages, "lapis" meaning stone and "lazuli" derived from the Arabic word for blue.

Latin cross: a cross with four arms in which the shorter transverse member crosses the upright one third from the top.

Lemel: the floor sweepings of precious metals from a jeweler's workshop.

Malachite: a copper carbonate mineral banded alternately bright and dark green. Because it polishes well and is opaque, it is excellent for carved flat brooches, pendants, and beads, and for a large variety

of objects and vessels.

Maltese cross: a cross with four arms of equal length and size, which widen as they extend from the center.

Marcasite: the trade name given to the tiny bright metallic stones called iron pyrites, when used in jewelry.

Memento Mori: for "Remember you must die." Jewelry intended as a reminder and warning of death, and reflecting this late 16th and 17th century preoccupation; featuring skulls and crossbones, skeletons, and coffins.

Moonstone: a silvery blue translucent stone generally cut en cabochon to display its silky sheen to best advantage.

Mussel pearls: or "River Pearls", produced by the freshwater mussel *Unio* found in some rivers of Europe and in the Mississippi Basin. Inferior to the oyster pearl.

Niobium: a rare, lustrous gray metal, similar in appearance to TITANIUM, though heavier and more expensive. Was extensively explored in the UK Nuclear Energy program. It is malleable and ductile so can be hand-worked, and this, together with its rich coloration on heating, has made it a popular metal with some jewelers today.

Obsidian: dark, glassy volcanic rock formed by rapid solidification of lava.

Onyx: a variety of CHALCEDONY, it is layered in shades of black and white, thus lending itself to cameo-cutting, the upper section forming a contrast with the lower.

Palmette: a fan-shaped decorative motif resembling a palm leaf.

Parkesine: the first polymer to be used commercially as a plastic and forerunner of CELLULOID. The invention of Alexander Parkes, it was introduced at the Great International Exhibition in London in 1862.

Parure (Fr.): a suite of matching jewelry. Also DEMI-PARURE, usually of two matching pieces only, e.g. necklace and earrings.

Paste: glass, usually containing lead oxide, which is used to simulate gemstones.

Pâte de Verre (Fr.): a glass-making technique in which crushed glass is made into a paste, colored with metallic oxides and fused. It is then molded and fired; the resulting glass is dense and opaque with a frosty surface.

Pavé, (pavé-set) (Fr.): a "paving" of stones, in which a number of small stones are set so closely together that the only discernible

fixing is the small metal grains which hold each stone in place.

Peridot: a transparent green gemstone popular since antiquity, it has a distinctive "oily" luster and has been used ceremonially in the past instead of emeralds.

Pinchbeck: an alloy of copper and zinc intended to simulate gold. Invented by the watchmaker Christopher Pinchbeck in the 18th century and used for making cheap jewelry set with pastes or inexpensive stones.

Platinum: recently discovered strong, silvery-white metal. It is more expensive than gold, neither corrodes nor tarnishes, but is very heavy. It has been used for jewelry since the 19th century.

Plique-à-Jour (Fr.): a technique of translucent enameling which, since it has no metal backing, allows light to travel through (hence *à jour*). The enamel is supported by a network of wire cells, and the effect is similar to stained glass.

Point cut: a polished diamond in its natural, octahedron, form. This very early style was superseded by later fashions.

Quartz: from *querertz* (Ger: "crossing ore") a reference to its tendency to run across other mineral veins. The most common of minerals, it is mostly crystalline. There are three varieties and many colours. See also ROCK CRYSTAL.

Reliquary: a richly decorated vessel or receptacle for a relic pertaining to the life or person of Christ or the saints.

Rhinestone: a type of ROCK CRYSTAL used as an inexpensive substitute for diamonds.

Rivière: a necklace consisting of single matched or graduated stones, usually diamonds.

Rock crystal: quartz in its natural state and quite colourless.

Rosary or Decade ring: a ring with 10 projections for counting the number of "Aves" to be said in each decade of the Rosary.

Rose-cut: a method of gemstone cutting with a flat base and a large number of triangular facets rising to a point.

Sardonyx: an ONYX banded alternately white and reddish-brown (Sard), often used for cameos and seals.

Sautoir (Fr.): a long necklace or chain sometimes enameled or jeweled, often worn diagonally across the body from shoulder to hip, or looped up and pinned

to the bodice or waistband. Also used to suspend spectacles or a watch.

Semiprecious stones: a term generally used to refer to all gemstones other than the PRECIOUS ones of diamond, ruby, emerald, sapphire, and pearl.

Sodalite: a mineral resembling LAPIS LAZULI, of which it is a component. It is also used as a gemstone in its own right.

Scarab: a type of beetle revered by the ancient Egyptians and used by them as an ornamental device, and for jewelry.

Scotch Pebble: the popular 19th-century name for the local Scottish AGATES and other HARDSTONES set into jewelry.

Table-cut: a method of gemcutting in which a square or rectangular "table" is cut on both the top and the bottom, the lower being smaller, and with four facets sloping upward and downward from the central "girdle."

Tiger's Eye: see CROCIDOLITE

Tinctured Doublet: a composite stone consisting of a layer of a precious stone cemented to a layer of an inferior one, which is also "tinctured" or dyed.

Titanium: a metallic element discovered in 1789, and used principally in aerospace technology. Now favored by some jewelers for the subtle and attractive range of colors it acquires when heated. It is also lightweight and durable.

Topaz: the so-called "yellow stone" which also occurs in a range of browns and as pale aquamarine. The rare pink variety (mostly obtained by heat treatment of brown stones) is highly prized.

Torc: a type of metal neck ring or armlet in the shape of an open hoop, often with ornamental terminals. Generally associated with Celtic jewelry.

Tourmaline: from the Sinhalese root meaning "colored stone," it possesses the widest color range of all the gemstones, resulting from its complex chemical composition. It can also be parti-colored.

Vinaigrette: a small decorative receptacle containing a sponge saturated in scented vinegar intended as an emergency treatment for faintness. Often worn on a chain suspended from a bracelet.

Yellow sapphire: sometimes known as "Oriental Topaz." it is a less valuable variety of the transparent "Corundum," of which the various blue sapphires are the most prized. Its color is due to ferric oxide.

187

INDEX

Page numbers in *italic* refer to the illustrations and captions

INDEX